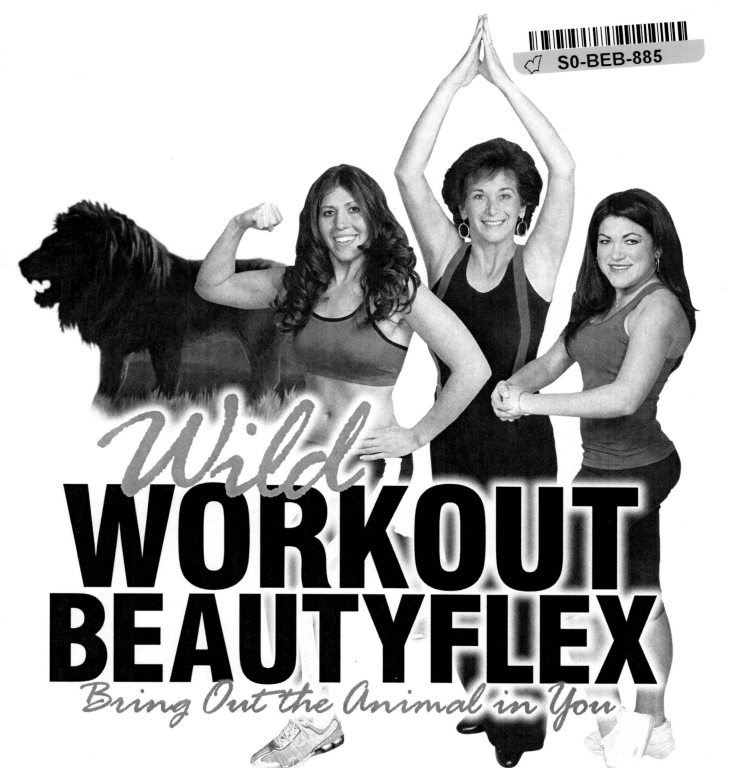

Wild WORKOUT BEAUTYFLEX
Bring Out the Animal in You

The FORYSTEKS'

LU Books
A Division of Liberty University Press

www.TheWildWorkout.com

S0-BEB-885

Wild WORKOUT BEAUTYFLEX

©2011 The Forysteks. All rights reserved.

No part of this publication may be reproduced or transmitted in any form or by any means, mechanical or electronic, including photocopying and recording, or by any information storage and retrieval system, without permission in writing from the author or publisher (except by a reviewer, who may quote brief passages and/or short brief video clips in a review.)

The scanning, uploading, and distribution of this book via the Internet or via any other means without the permission of the author or publisher is illegal and punishable by law. Please purchase only authorized electronic editions, and do not participate in or encourage electronic piracy of copyrighted materials. Your support of the author's rights is appreciated.

ISBN: 978-1-935986-08-9 Paperback

Published by:

LU
Books

LU Books
A Division of Liberty University Press
1971 University Blvd.
Lynchburg, VA 24551
www.liberty.edu/libertyuniversitypress

Cover Wrap Design by:
Megan Johnson

Interior Design and Layout by:
Heather Kirk

www.TheWildWorkout.com

NOTE: The exercises and advice contained within this book may be too strenuous and dangerous for some people, and the reader should consult their health practitioner before engaging in them. The information in this book is for educational purposes only. Neither the publisher nor author is engaged in rendering professional advice or services to the individual reader. All matters regarding physical and mental health should be supervised by a health practitioner knowledgeable in treating that particular condition. Neither the author nor the publisher shall be liable or responsible for any loss, injury, or damage allegedly arising from any information or suggestion in this book.

TABLE OF CONTENTS

FOREWORD

by Shari Falwell

"*And we know that all things work together for good to those who love God, to those who are the called according to **His** purpose.*" NKJV Sometimes in life we can't explain or understand why things happen the way they do. However, when it comes to control, I would much rather invest in my Heavenly Father's control than in my own. Trusting Him at His Word is where comfort, peace and joy can be found.

My friend, Julia Forystek, knows first hand what it's like to experience a life full of questions. As far as she could remember, her physical body worked differently than others. I'm sure there were many days when she wondered why she was "wired" the way that she was, but God had a plan and in that plan she put her entire trust. Now, years later, she uses her physical challenges to glorify her Creator who made her. Other individuals in the same position would more than likely "give up." But, Julia never did. Julia conquered what others would consider impossible. Now she uses her victory to help others. She is a success story and she never fails to give God the glory for using her in such a spectacular way.

In John 9, there is a story about the blind man whom the disciples were talking about to Jesus. I find that this illustration somewhat reflects what Julia has experienced in her life.

John 9:1-3 "*Now as Jesus passed by, He saw a man who was blind from birth. And His disciples asked Him, saying, 'Rabbi, who sinned, this man or his parents, that he was born blind?' Jesus answered, 'Neither this man nor his parents sinned, but that the works of God should be revealed in him.'*" NKJV

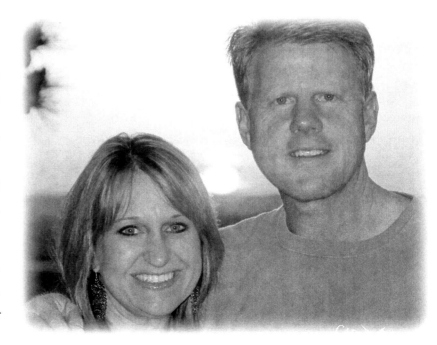

The NIV states, *"but this happened so that the work of God might be displayed in his life."*

The word, "Neither" shows that blame cannot be placed on Julia or her parents for why she was created this way. The latter part of the verse gives the answer that the physical issue had a purpose so the work of God could be "revealed" or "displayed." Julia is wanting to share with you the work of God in her life by "displaying" what she has learned through her experience. She wants you to share in the benefits that have not only made her physical body stronger but have made her spiritual body stronger than she ever dreamed possible.

Now, on a personal note, before I ever met Julia, I observed her from afar. Julia was a teacher at the academy where my children attended. She looked like she could be a student herself, but as I looked closer, I saw a beautiful young woman who carried herself with Christ-like confidence. And then as I watched her interact with others, she radiated and always appeared to be full of joy. Later, I found out her source of joy. It was Jesus.

I was able to share in music ministry with Julia later in our church. She loves to worship her Creator. Her worship continued throughout the week as she taught my older children truths from the Bible in middle school. Jonathan Jr., and Jessica have both shared with me on many occasions that Miss Forystek was their favorite Bible teacher. She encouraged growth! She made it fun, and challenging.

Julia has the gift of teaching. Now, she wants to invest in you! God has gifted her to help others spiritually and physically at the same time! I pray your investment in Wild Workout® proves beneficial. I've seen the results in Julia's entire family! It truly is amazing!

In closing, I want to go back to the verse I started with, Romans 8:28. *"And we know that all things work together for good to those who love God, to those who are the called according to His purpose."* NKJV

Julia, knows this verse is true, but there is a key word mentioned in the above and that word is "work". Lying around is not going to accomplish much physically or spiritually. It does take "work" to move forward and accomplish goals. You won't be sorry for "working" with Julia as she teaches you God given insights on how to make you feel better physically and spiritually.

Enjoy your "WORK!"

Shari Falwell

ACKNOWLEDGEMENTS

from Julia Forystek

*E*ver since I was a little girl my dad, Jim Forystek the creator of Wild Workout® instilled in me that my beauty lies within. He would teach me various Wild Workout® exercises and tell me that no matter what people or friends at school say, God has made me beautiful. I would look forward to his workout time because I would jump in and try to do the Wild Workouts® "just like daddy."

Gaining confidence from my dad, and thanking God for my body, led me to continue to do Wild Workout® to unveil my beauty that emulates from within! I am grateful that in college I was given the opportunity at Liberty University to join the all-women's traveling team called "True Identity." Through a variety of inspirational ways, True Identity encouraged teenage girls to throw away the lies, and believe that God has made them beautiful! My specialization was to speak on gaining self discipline, and taking care of the body for the Glory of God. I would also do various workouts with the young ladies to give them a chance to have fun, laugh, and enjoy learning how to beautify from within.

I had the privilege of working for the fitness program at Liberty University. I led a weekly Beauty-Flex® class which was primarily over taken by women. The ladies saw quick results and even wrote how much they enjoyed Wild Workout®. For example Patricia wrote,"…I really like how much we focused on ab work and leg work. It's good that we focus more on toning…Thanks so much Julia. Oh and these weekly goals are great. Thanks!"

Liberty University also featured its first Women's Fitness Seminar where I had the humbling privilege to open for our guest speaker. Together we got to teach the women a new way to workout.

My sister Jamee also went on to lead BeautyFlex® classes at LU. She inspires me with how she teaches others! Her fitness ability is awesome! When we were kids she loved to do one handed cartwheels around the front yard, laughing and making me smile! She still always reminds us to keep things simple, yet to challenge yourself and have fun. Jamee will teach you to be tough, and fit, and encourage you as she has me! She's my best friend, my sister, and I am so thankful to do BeautyFlex® with her.

My mom's stamina and energy still leaves me awestruck. She is up early every morning cooking healthy breakfast, and doing everything possible around the house. She would never settle for less than best and still doesn't. When we were kids I watched her with amazement as she cared for us five kids and I always asked if I could feel her arms because she had the strongest ones I knew. How else could she carry and hold us unless she possessed great strength.

I am thankful for Shari Falwell and her stance on equipping women with truth. Her dedication to encouraging women, including myself is so needed and appreciated! My hat goes off to her for all she does and supports in women's settings, groups, events and fitness.

I thank God for every single one of my students and all the kids I have been able to teach! Their smiles, spark, and amazing individual creativity is such a gift!

I am thankful for my family. They are closest to me, and know me best. They have provided friendship, perfect words for a moment in need, and accountability. For years we have done and enjoyed these exercises together and now you too can enjoy them with us. Wild Workout® is easy. It works with you, and with your schedule. You just have to put that first foot forward and start it. Let's get to it!

Your friend,

Julia Forystek

INTRODUCTION

*Y*our body is the most AWESOME invention God ever came up with! It builds itself, heals itself, repairs itself, and has a built-in heating and cooling system, an electrical power plant bursting with energy, a built-in defense system, and a central processing unit in the human brain that puts any computer to shame. Plus your body was designed to last a long time and feel good and healthy while being alive—the key is not just to add more years to your life but to add more life to your years! It is one of the only things in the universe that gets better the more you use it! Wow! It is truly awesome!

In today's society because of television, magazines, and billboards, women have a tendency to look at what other beautiful women possess and wish for it. Often times women continually wish, and therefore become unsatisfied with themselves, and ungrateful for the body given to them by their creator.

This is where the program BeautyFlex® comes in. BeautyFlex® uses God given power to beautify the body. It focuses the body's own resistance to develop it to its full potential.

BeautyFlex® is what women need today. Women are so busy yet still strive to be beautiful. This is why several eating disorders come about such as anorexia and bulimia, especially in college! Most women thrive on being thin and unfortunately think purging or starving themselves will give them their beauty they desire.

Ladies this is not the way!

What greater beauty is there than the beauty God has created? Animals reflect beauty because they are the way God has created them, and workout the way they were created to do so. This is the principle BeautyFlex® uses.

BeautyFlex® enhances YOUR body. Unlike other popular forms of exercise, Wild Workout® strengthens and shapes the body safely, without stressing the joints, connective tissues, and spine. Resistance is determined not by the weights on the bar or the setting on the machine, but by the BeautyFlexers own ability and desire to maintain resistance in the muscles as they work. Thus, BeautyFlex® not only develops strength, power, and endurance, but develops the ability to express these qualities through harmonious movement and with athletic grace.

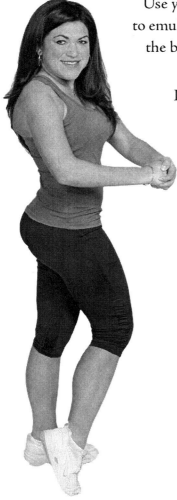

Use your own body to work for you rather than against you! Use Wild Workout® to emulate the beauty that lies within. You will feel better, and become satisfied with the body you were blessed with. Yes, YOUR BODY, not someone else's.

I have personally learned the benefits of fitness and it has changed my life. I will share more in detail with you later, but in a nutshell I learned to be thankful for the body I was given, and gratefully worked on it.

Ladies, be thankful for your body, and flex your inner beauty with Beauty Flex!!

WELCOME TO THE BEAUTIFUL WORLD OF WILD WORKOUT®

*T*hank you for choosing Wild Workout® BeautyFlex®, the total body workout program for women. As a woman, this program will work *with* you to transform and beautify your body quickly. Beauty Flex gives real results that you will be pleased with, and results without the use of steroids, drugs, weights, or expensive workout equipment. This program is based upon the same principles that build the most awesome, powerful, beautiful bodies within the animal kingdom.

The beauty of Wild Workout® is that it lets *you* start where *you* are, at *your* current level of fitness. You might be an on the go mom, an industrious college student, or a productive working woman but you *can* reach *your* fitness goals! If your goal is to be toned and sleek, with healthy muscle definition and shape, you can obtain that by the resistance you use for each exercise. **Fear not, you will not get big and bulky from doing these exercises.** You will become toned and elegant, allowing your clothes to flatter you. However, if you want more muscle development and definition on one area for whatever reason, put high resistance and muscle resistance into each movement while performing your Beauty-Flexes. If not, ease up on the level of resistance you put into each movement and exercise. Beautifying your body is simple with the Beauty Flex program, because it is coming from within you.

Letter from the creator of Wild Workout®, Jim Forystek

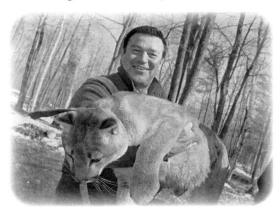

Welcome to the wonderful world of Wild Workout®. I commend you for having the courage to take the step that your body will reward you for an entire lifetime. It is always a great pleasure to know there are people such as you, who take control of their lives and health and go forward with confidence.

WORKOUT BEAUTYFLEX

Wild Workout® is the most revolutionary and powerful way to exercise for accelerated, powerful, eye-popping results. Yet the principle behind Wild Workout® is so simple. It is so simple and powerful, in fact, that mankind has overlooked it for centuries.

The most powerful, graceful, awe-inspiring, perfectly sculpted specimens of strength and beauty—the ones most appealing to the eyes and most inspiring to the imagination—aren't human beings, but animals. You see it clearly in the off-the-charts strength, exquisite grace, and royal beauty of the lion, which the Bible calls the strongest of beasts. It is also evident in the mesmerizing muscles and agility of the majestic elk that freely roams the upper elevations of the mountains as though child's play despite weighing over 1,000 pounds.

Yet when you consider the pillars of strength, the flexibility, the incredible speed, the ripped muscles, and the beauty of creatures among the animal kingdom, you'll notice there is no workout gym, no special equipment, no weights, no rowing machines, or dumbbells. It is all attained by using their body weight and energy and natural abilities.

It is this same principle that Wild Workout® is built upon, and make no mistake, it works—no ifs and buts. It's not up for questions or debate. The animals have already proven the point a million times, and it worked for me.

Based upon my physique alone, I was offered a full scholarship by the chancellor of a major East Coast college that turns out many professional football players. My chest muscles and upper body strength and overall look was gained through the Wild Workout® program, and the college chancellor was impressed. He wanted me on a plane within two days if I would be the fullback of their team.

I turned down the gracious offer, to pursue my Father's business, and I've turned down other offers since then. I've also coached and quarterbacked my own city league team to five championships and raised it to be one of the most feared and respected teams in the league. Because of Wild Workout® and the energy and glow and respectability it has given me as a person, I've grown accustomed to the notices, advances, and opportunities that come my way that others dream about.

Wherever I am, I am constantly approached and have doors opened for me by people who mistake me for a professional football player, an Olympic weightlifter, a bodybuilder, a professional wrestler, or an actor. My physique gets their attention, and they think that I must be someone special. Countless people have approached me and asked how many hours I spend in the gym a day, how much I bench press, and how I attained this level of physical fitness. Knowing that a proud arrogant braggart is the most unattractive person in the world, I usually respond to their inquiries by saying, "I'm on the George Foreman workout program—McDonalds for breakfast and Burger King for lunch."

Seriously, though, after you've sculpted your muscles, please feel free to tell your admirers that it's due to Wild Workout®.

Jim Forystek

HITTING THE BULL'S EYE

The Wild Workout® hits the bull's eye every time with your workouts—That's why you begin to see and feel results faster than you ever imagined possible! This is accomplished by TARGETING the area being worked and using the "Rifle" approach, we zero in on the bull's eye, put that area's muscles in the cross hairs of our scope and targeting specifically that area; we get a fantastic workout. The *Power Arrows* that accompany the illustrations shows you the direction in which to use resistance. If the **Power Arrow** is pointing up ↑ then resist on the upward motion, if the **Power Arrow** is Pointing Down ↓ then resist on the downward motion, and if the arrow in both directions resist going both directions. If there are no Power Arrows accompanying the illustration this means your body weight is all the resistance you need while performing this exercise (i.e. The Panther Flex I).

The amazing thing is, that as we see and feel results in that area very quickly we are also working many other muscle groups of our body at the same time, but because we are targeting a certain area and zeroing in on the bulls eye for that area for fast effective unbelievable results, the other muscles being worked are over shadowed but you start noticing results to the entire body.

For example our 1st BeautyFlex® the Panther Flex specifically targets the chest muscles, but as you're doing the Panther Flex even though it's hitting the bull's eye on the chest region, you're also at the same time bringing every muscle into play and giving them a workout your toes, your feet, your calves, your hamstrings, quads, glutes, abs, back, shoulders, neck, arms, hands, and fingers. So as you're specifically targeting the chest muscles and hitting the bull's eye seeing amazing results in that area, you're also getting a great workout in the rest of your body. We use the "rifle" approach to zoom in on the target and hit the bull's eye every time!!

Many people wonder why they've been working out for years and yet see no noticeable results, that's because other programs use the "shotgun" approach. Their shooting out a "spread" of BB's trying to hit everything and anything — and they end up hitting nothing. The Wild Workout® TARGETS the section we're working on and yes there is no question the target is a hit a direct Bulls Eye while also working other muscles. The BeautyFlex® workout is strategically laid out to bring you the most powerful workout EVER! While working the chest and bringing life giving oxygen to every muscle in the body, you're already preparing your abs for the next workout, while working the abs you're already preparing your neck and spine for the next workouts. While working the neck and spine you're already preparing the back. While working the back you're already preparing the legs, while working the legs you're already preparing the shoulders. While working the shoulders you're already preparing the arms, and when you get to the speed energy and endurance workout every muscle group that you've been through gets a phenomenal workout trying everything together. Plus when you move from one section to another, the section you're moving on from still comes into play as you begin your next workout so you never lose what you've just accomplished. It's AWESOME!!!

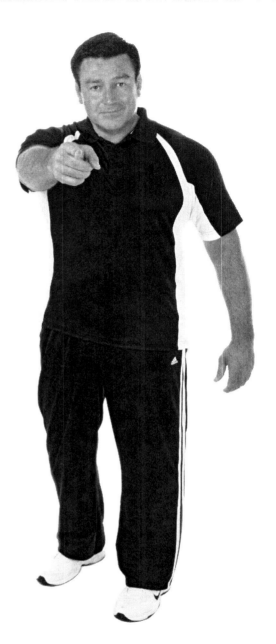

4 SECRETS OF HEALTH

*T*here are four secrets to health that are *so simple, yet so effective*—constantly refer to them, practice them, and make them part of your lifestyle, and you will be amazed at how easy it is to be and remain healthy! Being healthy is not found in trying out fad diets and chasing fancy and expensive trends. It is making solid healthy decisions on a consistent basis. Being healthy is a lifestyle, and when these four secrets become a part of your regular decisions, they will make all the difference in the world. Take them seriously and make them a part of your life starting today.

SECRET #1—EXERCISE

The human body was created to last a long time. It's one of the only things in the universe that gets BETTER the more you use it! Experts agree that exercise will help:

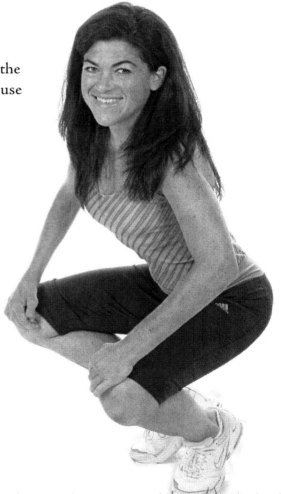

- **Keep your weight under control**
- **Reduce your risk of heart disease, diabetes, and high blood pressure**
- **Improve your blood cholesterol levels**
- **Prevent bone loss**
- **Boost your energy levels**
- **Manage tension**
- **Improve self-image**
- **Control anxiety**
- **Control depression**

Exercise on a regular basis. The only things that don't move are rocks and the dead! Exercise regularly. You now have BeautyFlex®, which can be done anywhere at anytime, so NO EXCUSES!

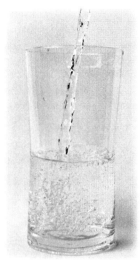

SECRET #2—DRINK ENOUGH PURE WATER EVERY DAY

Experts agree that our bodies require a minimum of at least eight glasses of pure water a day. If you are very active and involved in strenuous exercise, you should drink much more than that. After all, seventy percent of your body is made up of water—not protein, not carbs, not meat, or anything else. PURE WATER is liquid life. Through daily sweating, breathing, carrying oxygen to muscles, helping to digest food, flushing waste products from the body, lubricating joints, and *so* much more, *so* much of our water is lost daily. Even if you are a couch potato, your water level must be replenished—eight glasses a day minimum.

The next time you are at the store, and your hand is reaching for a soda, say, "No. I will grab a water drink instead." It is now available everywhere in a variety of forms—spring, artesian, natural, bottled at source, carbonated, flavored with pure fruit juices, in a bottle, in a can, by the gallon, six pack, case—at the office, delivered to your home in five-gallon jugs. It's everywhere. So there is no excuse to not pass on the soda and sugar drinks and drink eight glasses of pure water a day. It's more important than your diet. Because seventy percent of you is water, give yourself a break and drink some!

SECRET #3—STAY AWAY FROM WHITE BREAD, WHITE SUGAR, AND WHITE FLOUR

Experts agree that there are many healthier choices than "white" foods:

> **White bread**—rather, choose whole wheat, whole grain, rye, pumpernickel, multigrain, etc.
>
> **White sugar**—rather, choose honey, brown sugar, unprocessed cane sugar, etc.
>
> **White flour**—rather, choose whole wheat noodles, spinach noodles, brown rice, etc.

It's the processing, bleaching, etc. of the white products that make them an unwise choice. Many people have pounds and pounds of waste stuck in their intestines because of their poor diet of these types of foods—plus they are clogged!

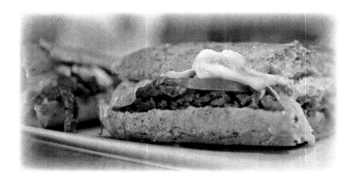

The healthy choices are not only good for you and add nutrients to your body, but they also help to keep you clean inside and properly cleansed within. The healthy choices are everywhere and conveniently available from supermarkets to restaurants. So no excuses—choose healthy.

Ask for a whole wheat bun for your burger. Yes, the fast food places will give you one. You only have to ask. Ask for whole wheat noodles with your pasta. Ask for spinach noodles, ask for honey, ask for a whole wheat crust in your pizza. Get your sandwich on multigrain bread. You have not because you ask not! No excuses!

SECRET #4—EAT BAKED, NOT FRIED

Experts agree that the frying of foods is what soaks everything full of grease, fat, and lard! Go for a baked potato, not French fries. Go for baked chips, not fried. Go for baked, grilled, broiled, or flame-broiled lean meat, fish, turkey, steak, or chicken—anything but fried and deep fried.

Use virgin olive oil instead of lard. It's your choice. Make it—no excuses! Plus you can snack all you want, if you snack on the right healthy foods.

Here's a list to help you:

FRUITS

Apples	Oranges
Plums	Kiwi
Coconut	Nectarines
Tangerines	Berries
Strawberries	Raspberries
Melons	Grapefruit
Grapes	Bananas

VEGETABLES

Cauliflower	Broccoli
Carrots	Green peppers

Lettuce	Cucumbers
Peas	Beets
Celery	Cabbage
Green beans	Radishes

RAW NUTS and SEEDS

Sunflower seeds	Almonds
Cashews	Walnuts
Hazel nuts	Brazilian nuts
Hickory nuts	Peanuts in the shell

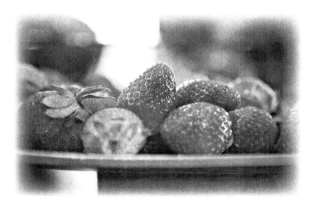

Just be careful you are not loading up your snack choices with fattening sauces and dips and that the seeds and nuts are not coated with salt or candied. Every grocery store now has a wide selection of these healthy snacks, so go load up on them. Leave your excuses behind!

3 MOTIVATION TIPS THAT WORK

*M*y friend, be prepared to face the fact that there will be days when you flat out won't want to exercise. You just won't feel like it. Here are three fantastic tips that will overcome that deflated feeling and get you to exercise anyway, and you will be so glad you did. These work, so use them!

MOTIVATION TIP #1

Have a set of exercise clothes that are for the exclusive purpose of wearing when you exercise and for nothing else—not for knocking around the house, not for going out in public. The only purpose of these clothes is for exercise. I have many sets of shorts, T-shirts, and tank tops that I only wear when exercising.

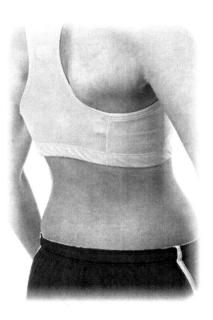

Why? What you wear determines how you act. When wearing an evening gown, you don't feel much like playing tackle football. When wearing your favorite ripped jeans and T-shirt with your comfortable tennis shoes, you don't feel much like standing around in church. What you wear determines your mind-set, and when you are having one of those days when you're looking for an excuse to not exercise, go put your exercise clothes on. Your mind-set will begin to change.

MOTIVATION TIP #2

Turn on your favorite music and crank it up! When you think you have it loud, give it another boost even louder. Push the volume to the verge of being obnoxious. Your favorite music blasting will begin to overcome your deflated feeling, your mood will shift gears, and your attitude will change. Even little babies can't keep still when they hear good music—they begin to smile, bounce up and down, and move

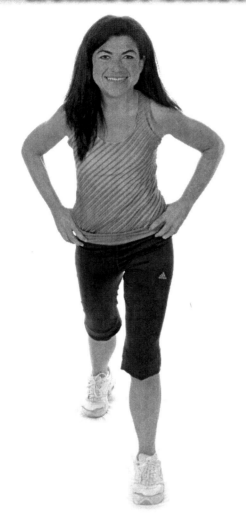

to the beat. Use that power of music for yourself, and your motivation will greatly surprise you!

MOTIVATION TIP #3

The human body is so advanced you can't begin to comprehend how great it is. Your body is already programmed to fill in the gaps. Whenever you watched a movie, you might have thought you saw all the action and movement, but you actually only saw still pictures, and your mind filled in the gap between them to make them appear in full action. That's why subliminal messages were outlawed from movies, because even though they were too fast for a person's eye to see, people's minds saw them, and they were affected.

Theaters used to flash soda or popcorn ads during movies, and people would get thirsty or want popcorn. Even though their eyes didn't see them, their minds picked up on the images. Use this advanced knowledge to your advantage. When you don't feel like exercising, tell yourself, "Well, I'll get my exercise clothes on, crank up my music, and I'll exercise. But I'm going to take it slow. I'm not going to break any records. I'm not going to push myself today. I'll take it easy and just get them done."

When you start to do your workouts during these times, you'll find you have some of your very best workouts. You get started, take the pressure off by telling yourself you are just going to take it easy, and your body takes over and fills in the gaps. When you're done, you'll smile and say, "Wow! That was an awesome workout. I'm glad I did it!" Put on your exercise clothes. Crank up the music. Tell yourself you're not going to break any records today. These helpful hints will get you over the hump! Use them! No excuses!

OUR MISSION

"Wild Workout® BeautyFlex® is dedicated to empowering women to be thankful for the body that was given to them and to improve it. To build health, and fitness naturally by using their body's own energies and abilities—as the creatures of the animal kingdom do."

Workout Rotation

To get started with Wild Workout®, it is recommended that you rotate the sets of exercises that concentrate on different muscle groups in this fashion:

Week 1: Chest Workout only

Week 2: Chest and Abdominal Workouts

Week 3: Chest, Spine, and Neck Workouts

Week 4: Chest and Back Workouts

Week 5: Chest and Leg Workouts

Week 6: Chest and Shoulder Workouts

Week 7: Chest and Arm Workouts

Week 8: Chest and Speed, Energy, and Endurance Workouts

The Chest Workout is critical to do all eight weeks of this course. This is because the BeautyFlexes in the Chest Workout will force you to breathe deeply, which will trigger muscle growth and development throughout your body. You will also be pleased with what it does for your womanly figure.

Once you've completed the entire course, you can go through the entire course again. If you feel one area needs more work than the other you can repeat the cycle again, if you wish. Or you can replace the Chest Workout with one of the other Workouts, rotating the other Workouts weekly for eight weeks until you've done them all.

Another option is to build your own routine by choosing one exercise from each Workout. Since each of the Workouts in this course contains five BeautyFlexes, you have a wide variety to choose from to prevent boredom as you continue to develop your body.

Building your own routine allows you to focus on problem areas. For example, if you want to focus on your abdominals, do the whole Abdominal Workout during every session, along with at least one BeautyFlex® from each of the other Workouts. Your routine would look like this:

- **Dolphin Flex I**
- **Dolphin Flex II**
- **Shark Flex I**
- **Shark Flex II**
- **Dolphin Flex III**
- **A Chest Exercise**
- **A Spine Exercise**
- **A Neck Exercise**
- **A Back Exercise**
- **A Leg Exercise**
- **A Shoulder Exercise**
- **An Arm Exercise**
- **A Speed, Energy, and Endurance Exercise**

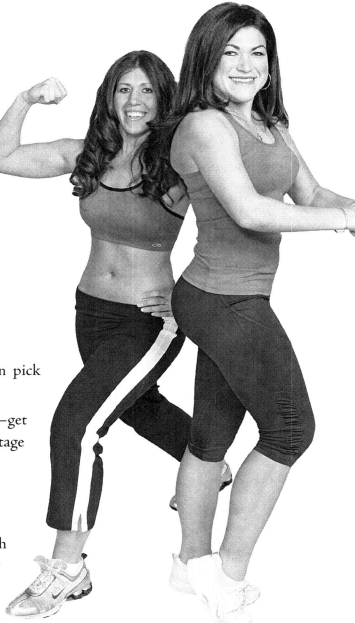

Follow this routine for as long you want, then pick another area to focus on and begin again.

It's your body to beautify, and the sky's the limit—get creative and use Wild Workout® to your best advantage to bring out the beauty you posses!

Number of Repetitions

Along with instructions for performing each BeautyFlex® in this course, there is a listed number of repetitions to do, based on how advanced a

BeautyFlexer is. Level One is for beginners; Level Two is for intermediate trainees, and Level Three is for advanced trainees.

Whether you're new to regular exercise or are already fit from other activities, you shouldn't go beyond Level One during your first week of training. If you can't do the number of repetitions listed for Level One, that's fine—begin your journey where you are. As you do each BeautyFlex®, concentrate on the muscles that particular BeautyFlex® is designed to work, and remember train, don't strain!

It's a good idea to log your workouts in your BeautyFlex® Journal. Writing down the BeautyFlexes and the number of repetitions you do gives you a record of your progress.

Workout Tip: Performing your BeautyFlexes in front of a full-length mirror and wear clothing that lets you see your muscles working. Watching yourself while BeautyFlexing will help you use proper technique. As you do each BeautyFlex®, try to concentrate on the muscles that you are working, this will help you get a much better workout. For example, as you do Gorilla Flex IV (the first bicep BeautyFlex® in the Arm Workout), focus your eyes on your biceps as your arm flexes and extends.

Workout Frequency

Some people do two or three Wild Workout® sessions per week. But if you want to see quick improvement, I recommend working out at least five times per week.

Wild Workout® can be done anywhere, anytime, and don't require special equipment. You could even BeautyFlex® five times per week while watching your favorite half-hour TV show and finish your workout before the show ends!

Whether you work out five, three, six, or two days per week, what matters most is that you're consistent, week in and week out. Stick with it and don't quit! No excuses! Your body will thank you for it a million times over!

You *are* beautiful! Use Wild Workout® BeautyFlex® and bring out your inner beauty!

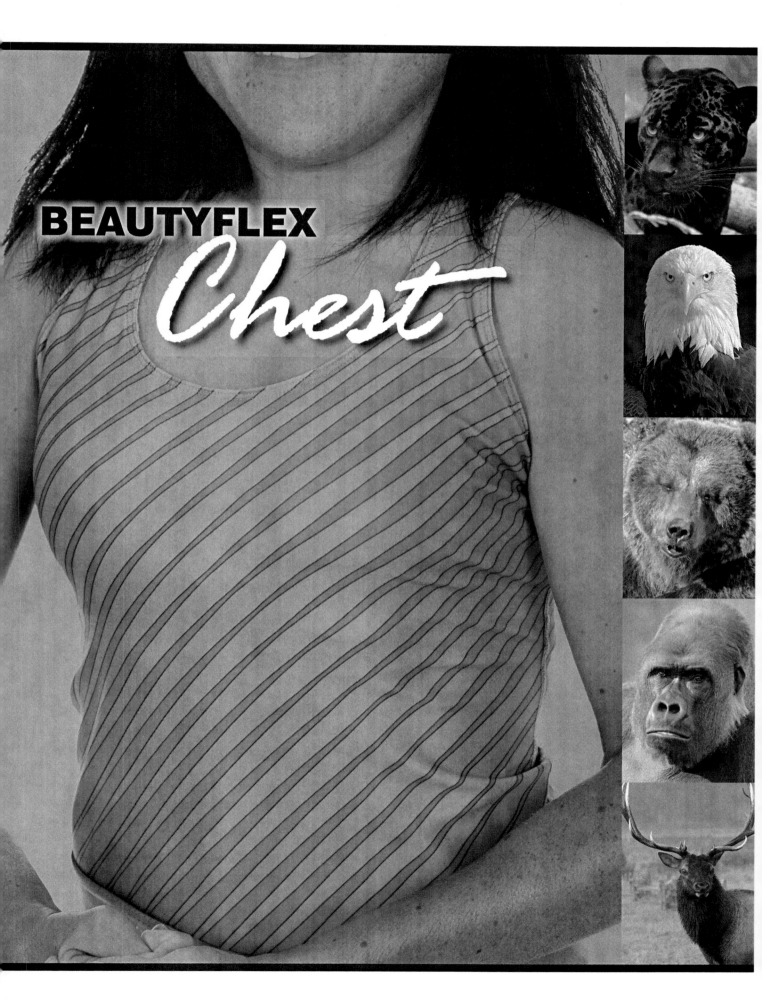

BEAUTYFLEX *Chest*

CHEST WORKOUT

*T*he Wild Workout® program for building a well developed, feminine upper body, without special equipment, is based on God's beautiful animals that possess chest strength—the panther, eagle, bear, gorilla, and elk. All you need are 5 simple BeautyFlexes, 20 minutes per day, and your own best effort!

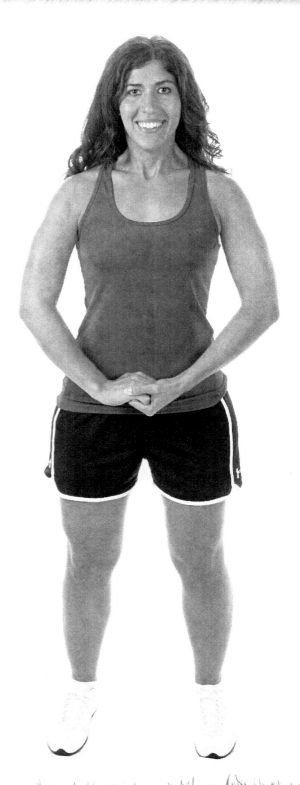

#1—PANTHER FLEX I

*W*e have all heard the timeless analogy of the old lady and her many cats. Regardless of the negative connotation sometimes attached, women have a special relationship with such beautiful creatures. Ironically enough the first chest BeautyFlex® is the Panther Flex. When a panther or any member of the cat family gets ready to strike their prey, they crouch and flex their massive chest muscles that give them such extraordinary leaping ability as they spring upon their mark. The Panther Flex stimulates that flex for the chest. We have all done push-ups from time to time—well now get ready to take the humble push-up to the next level.

To do the Panther Flex, do push-ups between two chairs (or any sturdy objects of equal height). Set your chairs just a little wider than shoulder-width apart and let your body sink a little lower than the chairs as you go down. It's this extra flex that feeds and nourishes and works your chest muscles. Don't be fooled, this BeautyFlex® *will* give you the results you are looking for.

> **LEVEL THREE: 50 repetitions**
> **LEVEL TWO: 20 repetitions**
> **LEVEL ONE: 5-10 repetitions**

If you are a little sore the next day, feel free to break up your repetitions into sets. For example instead of doing 50 all at once, do five sets of ten, with breaks in between. Also be sure you are drinking plenty of water. Experiment to see what works for you and do not do more than you are comfortable with.

What matters most is that you do your BeautyFlexes consistently—day after day, week after week, month after month. You will not have long to wait, though, before your consistency and patience start to reap their rewards.

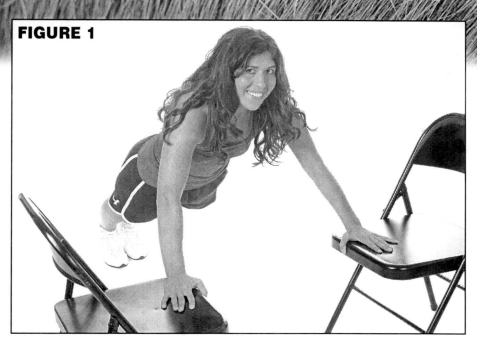

FIGURE 1

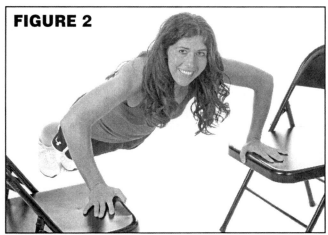

FIGURE 2

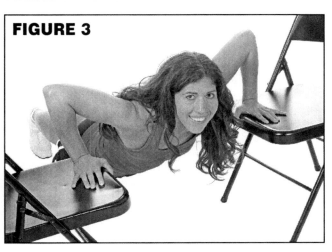

FIGURE 3

Modified

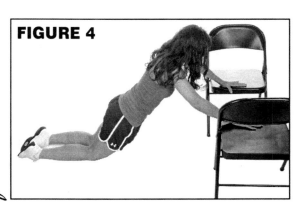

FIGURE 4

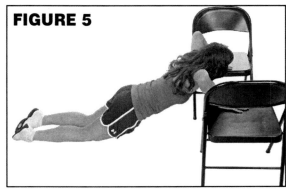

FIGURE 5

#2—EAGLE FLEX I

The eagle is the symbol of one of the greatest countries on earth. It also represents rising up and overcoming problems—soaring, regardless of your circumstances. An eagle's broad wings carry it to great heights—even above the highest mountaintops. The eagle's ability to such strength is its incredible chest muscles which flex each time it flaps its wings.

To perform the Eagle Flex, stand straight up with your feet shoulder-width apart and your arms straight down at your sides. Slowly raise your arms, keeping them straight as an eagle's wing, while flexing your chest muscles. Reach and extend farther as you raise your arms and extend them as wings. Extend them until your hands are just a little higher than your head, then bring your arms in front of you crossing them at the top, as you bring your arms down, flex, pushing up with one, and down with the other. Breathe—fill your lungs—and exhale as you come down. Alternate which arm you place on top.

This exercise develops the chest muscles quickly, and the deep breathing it involves will stimulate muscle growth throughout your body.

LEVEL THREE: 35 repetitions
LEVEL TWO: 20 repetitions
LEVEL ONE: 10 repetitions

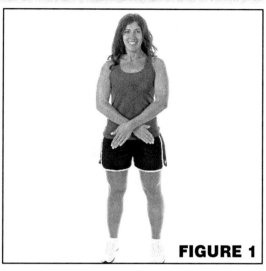

FIGURE 1

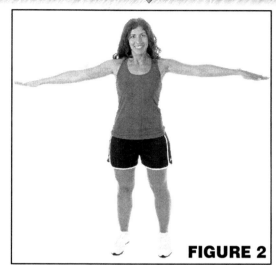

FIGURE 2

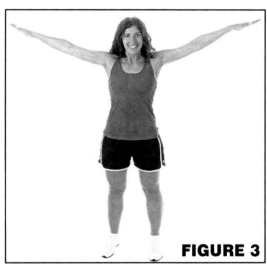

FIGURE 3

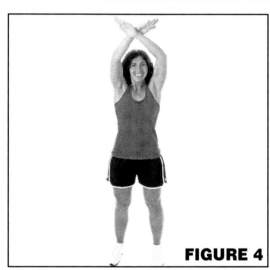

FIGURE 4

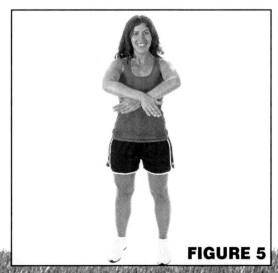

FIGURE 5

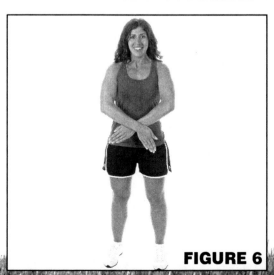

FIGURE 6

#3—BEAR FLEX I

a simple hug can bring a smile to a woman's face, and can take her breath away all at the same time. A bear hug on the other hand, if given in full force can literally take ones breath away, and might not quite be the loving embrace one was hoping for. The bear is admired and feared for its ability to tightly grasp other creatures. The Bear Flex I simulates a bear hug.

Stand with your hands in front of you, a little lower than your waist. With one hand turned up and the other turned down, grip and interlock your fingers in a cupped position. With your fingers locked and pulling apart, slowly lift your hands while keeping them close to your body until your hands are over your head, flexing your chest muscles as you do it. Keep the tension on, pulling apart with fingers interlocked. Then slowly move back down to the starting position.

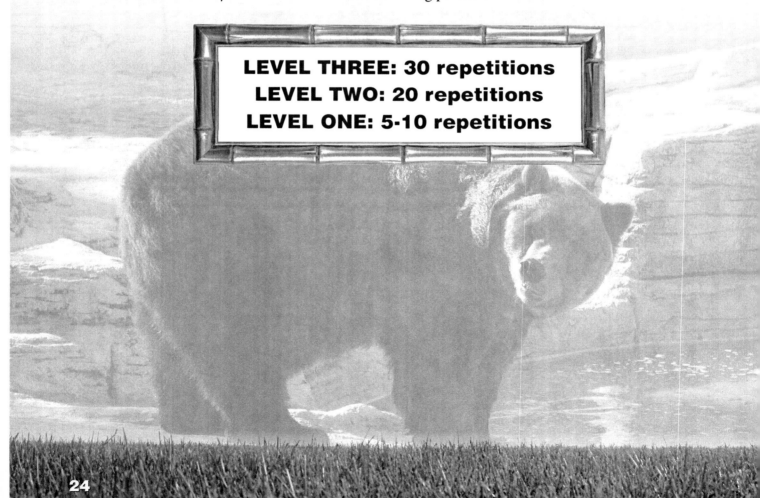

LEVEL THREE: 30 repetitions
LEVEL TWO: 20 repetitions
LEVEL ONE: 5-10 repetitions

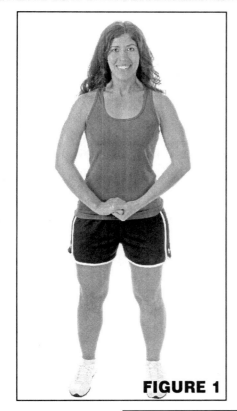

FIGURE 1

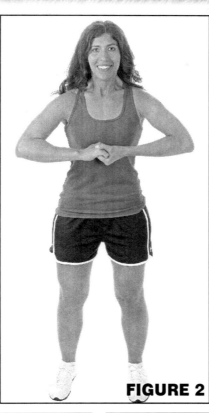

FIGURE 2

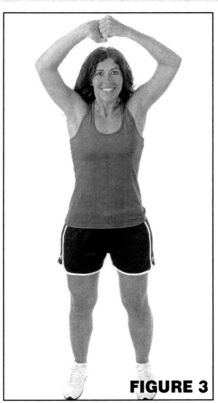

FIGURE 3

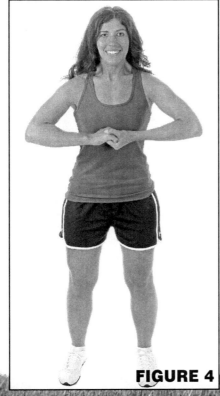

FIGURE 4

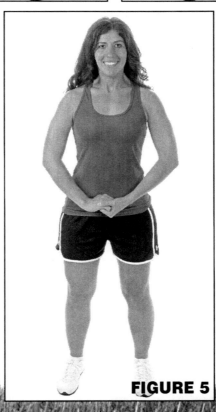

FIGURE 5

#4—GORILLA FLEX I

*T*he massive gorilla pounds proudly on his immense chest to display his superiority. Does this remind you of any men you have previously dated? As a woman you might not want the gorilla's intimidating strength, but nonetheless you cannot ignore the size of their chest, and firmness it possess. Regardless of their size, gorillas display mind-boggling strength and agility as they swing and climb on vines and branches. Fortunately, you don't need vines, branches, or special equipment to simulate this chest firming movement, thanks to the Gorilla Flex I.

Imagine there's a climbing rope hanging in front of you. Standing with your feet shoulder-width apart, grab that imaginary rope, clinch it in your fists tightly in front of you just above your head. Then flex your chest muscles as you slowly pull that rope down. Flex, pull, and grip with each hand, until both hands are a bit lower than your waist. Raise your hands above your head again, alternate your other hand on top and repeat.

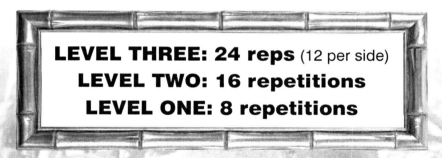

LEVEL THREE: 24 reps (12 per side)
LEVEL TWO: 16 repetitions
LEVEL ONE: 8 repetitions

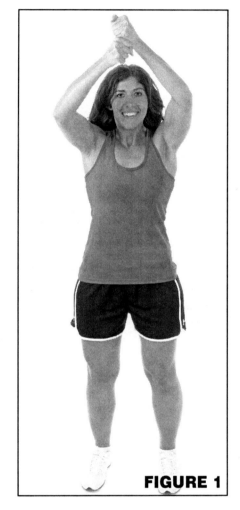

FIGURE 1

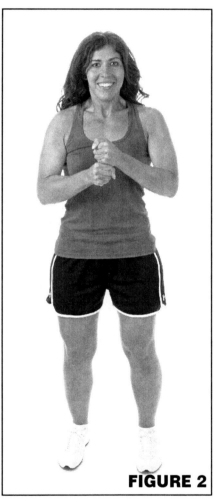

FIGURE 2

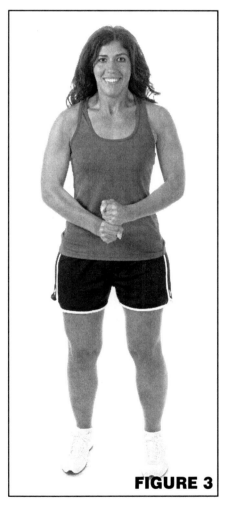

FIGURE 3

#5—BULL ELK FLEX I

*O*ne glimpse of a bull elk in the wild is enough to make the strongest heart feel faint! The female protects her young by proudly standing over it displaying her strong chest with posture. She possesses powerful lungs that allow her to climb mountaintops at over 10,000 feet with ease. Nothing will stand in her way when it comes to her young. The Bull Elk Flex I brings into play the working of the elk's muscles as he resists and flexes to climb the tallest mountain.

Make a fist with one hand and place the fist in the palm of the other hand, with your knuckles on the palm and the inside of the fisted hand close to your body. Keep your upper arms straight at your sides, slightly ahead of you, bending only at the elbows. Start with the palm of the hand about chest high, then push down on that palm with your fist, resisting the fist with the palm and flexing your chest muscles, just as a bull elk goes up a mountainside. Slowly allow the fist to overcome the palm, forcing the arm down slowly until it is a little lower than your waist. Now do the same exercise on the other side, reversing the position of your hands.

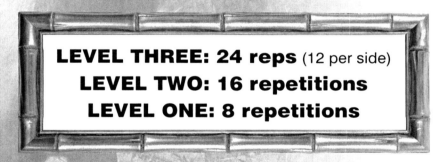

LEVEL THREE: 24 reps (12 per side)
LEVEL TWO: 16 repetitions
LEVEL ONE: 8 repetitions

Performing these five BeautyFlexes with consistency, determination, and patience will earn you the chest development you desire. Remember to breathe deep, and keep good posture. It won't be long before you see the fruit of your labors. Not only will your body improve, but your health, and self confidence as well. My friend, women are social beings so please feel free to call, write, or email me and let me know how you are progressing. I want to rejoice in your progress with you!

However far along you are with Wild Workout®, I want to commend you again for your determination to improve your fitness, appearance, and health—to "walk the walk," not just "talk the talk"!

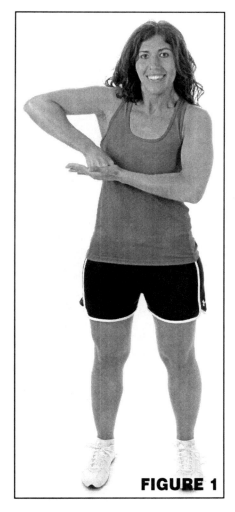

FIGURE 1

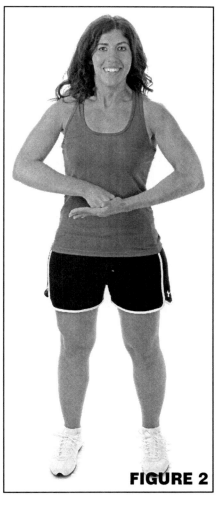

FIGURE 2

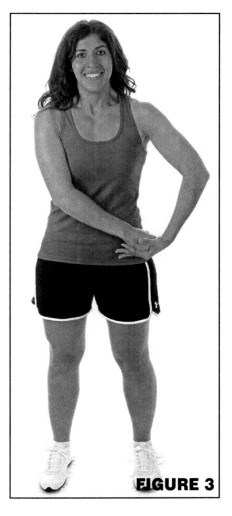

FIGURE 3

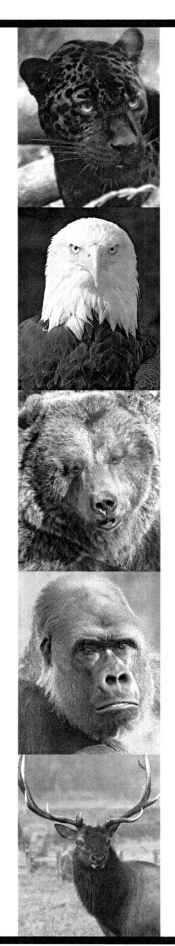

Chest Exercises

PANTHER FLEX I

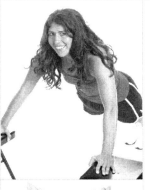

EAGLE FLEX I

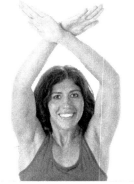

BEAR FLEX I

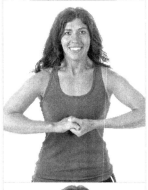

GORILLA FLEX I

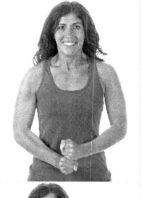

ELK FLEX I

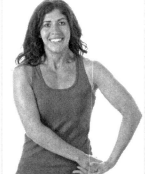

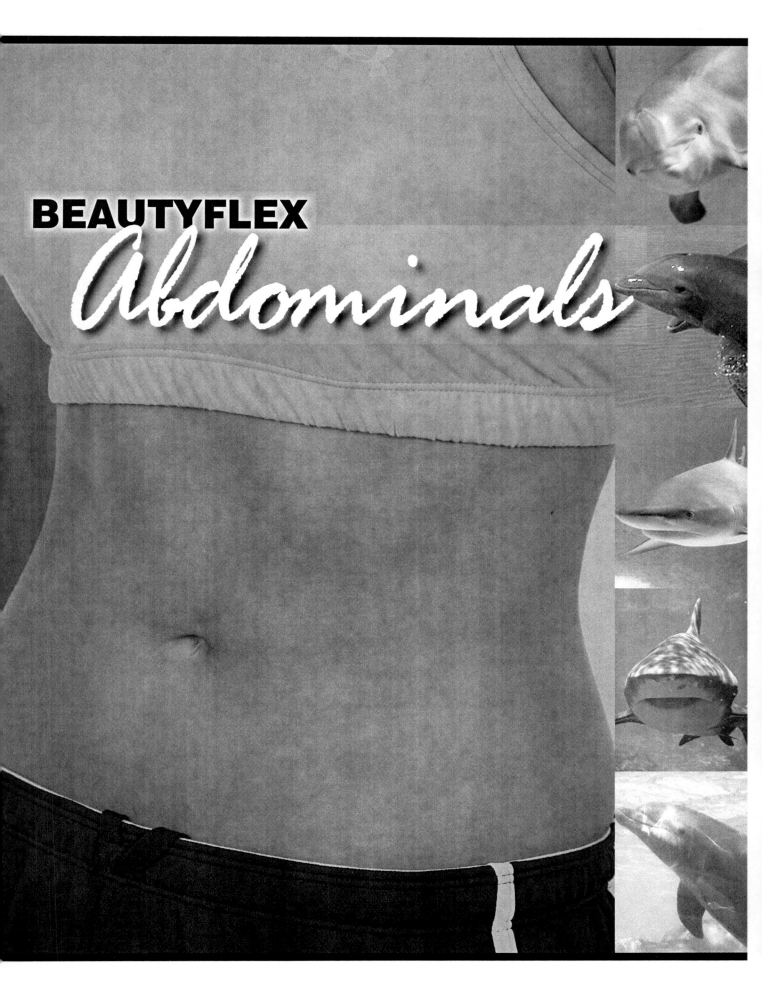

BEAUTYFLEX *Abdominals*

THE BEST IS NEVER OVER

The best is never over,
The best has never gone,
There's always something lovely
To keep you struggling on.

There's always compensation,
For every cross you bear,
A secret consolation,
Hidden well somewhere.

Ends are new beginnings,
As one day you will see;
The best is never over,
The best is yet to be!

Author: Unknown

ABDOMINALS WORKOUT

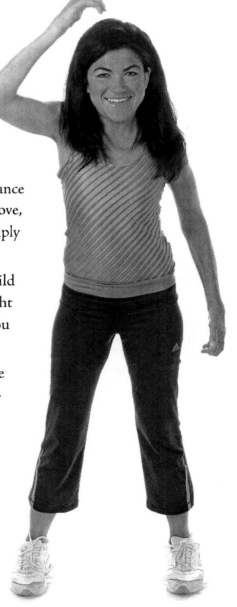

*Y*ou can have a flat, sleek, and sexy stomach! No equipment, weights, pulleys, or machines! Just five simple BeautyFlexes for 20 minutes a day.

Wild Workout® for a Flat, Sleek, and Toned Stomach

A well defined chest combined with a flat sexy stomach will enhance what is already there, you're a knockout! Allow your confidence to improve, and tell yourself you have the strength to overcome circumstances simply because you have improved what you already had in you!

With consistency, determination, and patience, it is possible to build strong, well-defined abdominal muscles more quickly than you might have thought. Strengthening your abdominal muscles will help you breathe more deeply, too, which will improve your general health.

No earthly creatures that I know of have stronger, more impressive abdominal muscles than the dolphin and the shark. Imagine the incredible strength it takes for a trick-show dolphin to pull itself out of the water and "walk" across it by balancing on its tail and flexing its abdominal muscles! Talk about functional strength! Sharks, on the other hand, don't do cute tricks for tourists. Their power, speed, and ferocity have inspired respect and terror for many years. Now let's bring out more beauty with Wild Workout®!

#1—DOLPHIN FLEX I

*D*olphins swim by using their abdominal muscles to move their tail fins up and down. This Beauty-Flex® imitates that movement.

Lie flat on the floor on your back (or on an exercise mat or carpet). Put your hands under your buttocks with your palms down. Your legs should be together and straight. Keeping your legs together and straight, lift them until they're pointing straight up. Then lower them to the floor again.

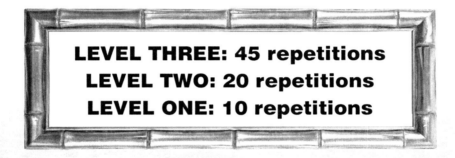

LEVEL THREE: 45 repetitions
LEVEL TWO: 20 repetitions
LEVEL ONE: 10 repetitions

Remember: do only as many repetitions as you can do comfortably.

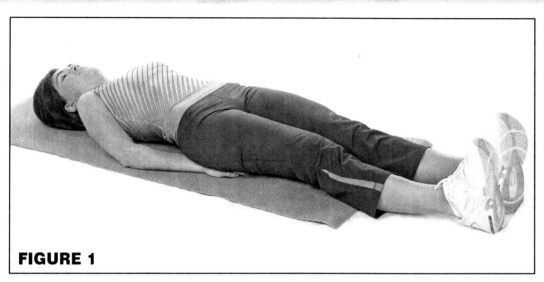

FIGURE 1

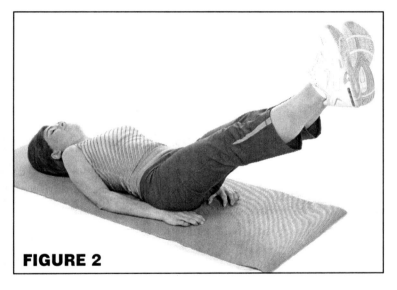

FIGURE 2

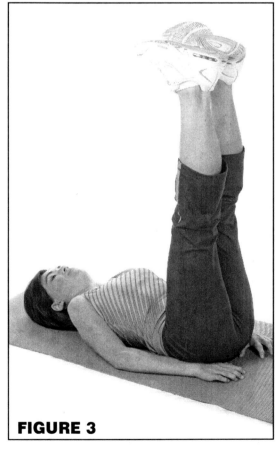

FIGURE 3

#2—DOLPHIN FLEX II

*L*ie flat on the floor on your back (or on an exercise mat or carpet). Keep your legs together and straight, resting the palms of your hands beside your ears. Tense your abdominal muscles, pushing your belly button into the floor, and sit up as far as you can while keeping your legs on the floor. Do not strain your back. Look up at the ceiling, and bring your chin up first. Try to touch your elbows to your knees. If you can, great. If you can't, that's okay—raise your body as far as you can without straining. This stimulates the stomach muscles, similar to the dolphin's movements.

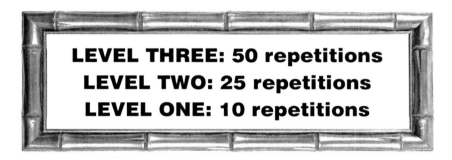

LEVEL THREE: 50 repetitions
LEVEL TWO: 25 repetitions
LEVEL ONE: 10 repetitions

This BeautyFlex® is tough for most woman—but then again, "most women" will not do the work necessary to build a beautiful abdomen. Patience and consistency are your keys. Exercise is like a bank account: you only get out of it what you put into it. And when you put a lot into it, expect to earn interest!

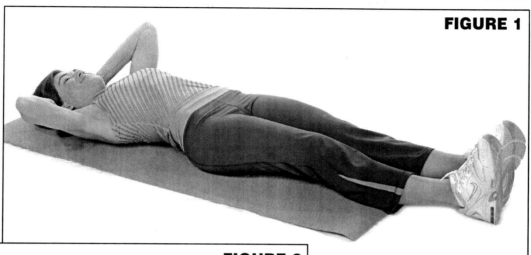

FIGURE 1

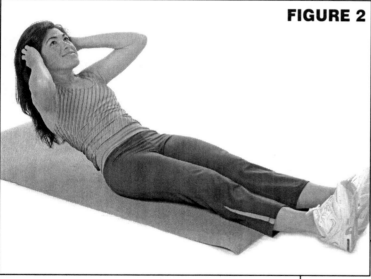

FIGURE 2

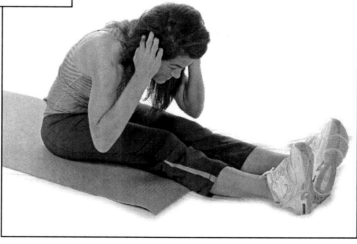

FIGURE 3

#3—SHARK FLEX I

*D*olphins swim by moving their tails up and down, but it was observed by the creator of Wild Workout® that sharks swim by moving their tails from side to side. You need to do both up-and-down and side-to-side movements to strengthen your abdominal muscles from all angles.

Lie flat on the floor on your back (or on an exercise mat or carpet). Put your hands under your buttocks with your palms down. Lift your legs until they point straight up. Now, move your feet like the shark moves its fins. Open your legs until they form a wide V, then bring them back together and cross them. Your right foot will stretch toward the left and your left foot will stretch toward the right. It's a four-part movement: up, out, cross, and down. With each repetition, alternate which leg you cross in front.

LEVEL THREE: 40 repetitions
LEVEL TWO: 20 repetitions
LEVEL ONE: 10 repetitions

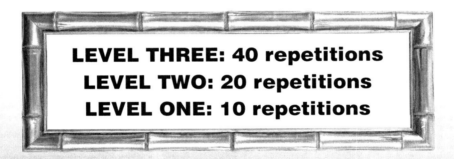

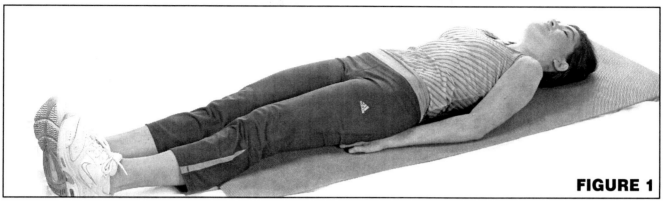

FIGURE 1

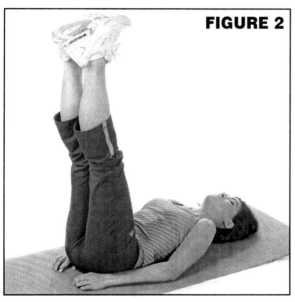

FIGURE 2

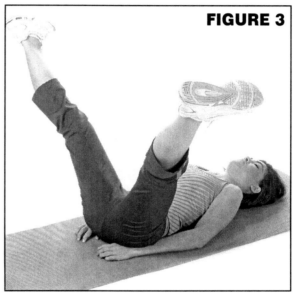

FIGURE 3

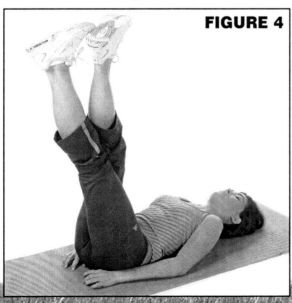

FIGURE 4

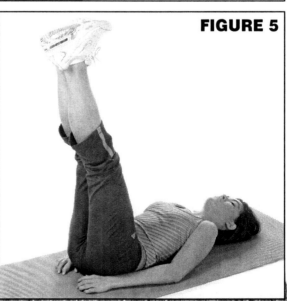

FIGURE 5

#4—SHARK FLEX II

*S*ome women have said they would like to take a little "love" out of their handles. This BeautyFlex® targets the obliques, the muscles underneath those "love handles." You are going to simulate the shark's side-to-side movement with your upper body.

Stand with your hands on your hips, your feet shoulder-width apart, and your legs straight. Bend to your right as far as you can without straining. Let your right hand slide down your right leg as you bend. As your right hand slides down, curl your left arm upward until it's over your head and pointing to the right. Doing this will help you bend a little farther to the right. Return to the starting position and repeat, bending to your left this time.

LEVEL THREE: 50 reps (25 per side)
LEVEL TWO: 30 repetitions
LEVEL ONE: 20 repetitions

Again, don't stretch farther than is comfortable for you. Remember: BeautyFlexes should feel good to do!

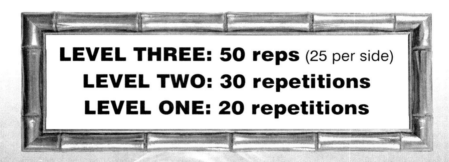

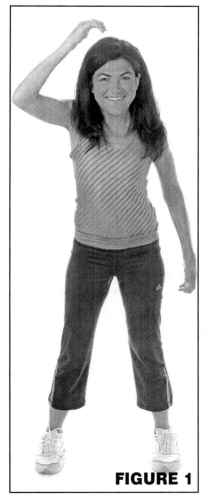

FIGURE 1

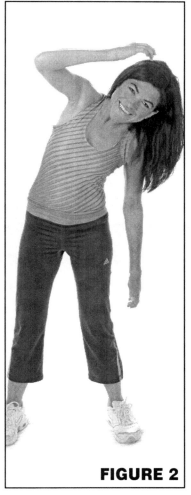

FIGURE 2

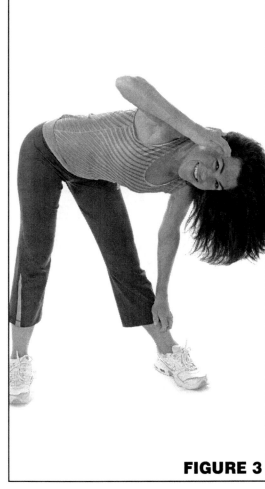

FIGURE 3

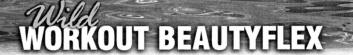
#5—DOLPHIN FLEX III

*H*ere is one last up-and-down movement to finish your workout. First, set a sturdy chair or stool a few feet away from a heavy piece of furniture (such as a bed, dresser, or couch). Sit sideways on the chair or stool and slide your feet under the bed, dresser, or couch.

Now that you are in position, rest the palms of your hands beside your ears and lean back slowly. If you can, lean back until your body's parallel to the floor. Then tense your abdominal muscles as you sit back up.

Don't lean back farther than is comfortable for you.

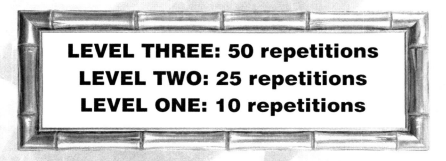

LEVEL THREE: 50 repetitions
LEVEL TWO: 25 repetitions
LEVEL ONE: 10 repetitions

That, my friend is the Wild Workout® stomach workout. By practicing these five BeautyFlexes regularly and eating sensibly, you will build lean abs where your belly used to be! Just to be clear, "eating sensibly" means eating lots of fresh vegetables and fruits, along with whole grains and lean meat. Again, be sure to drink plenty of water, too.

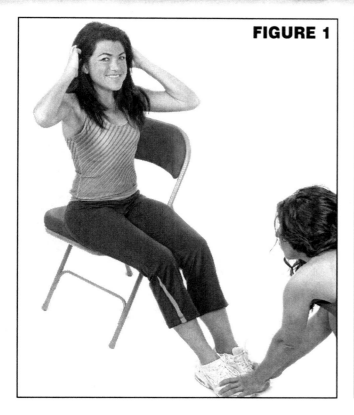

FIGURE 1

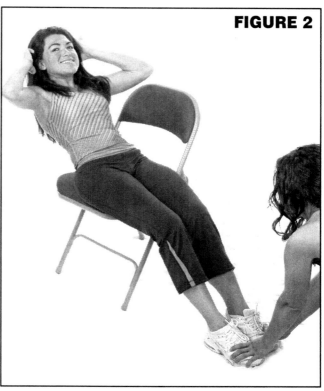

FIGURE 2

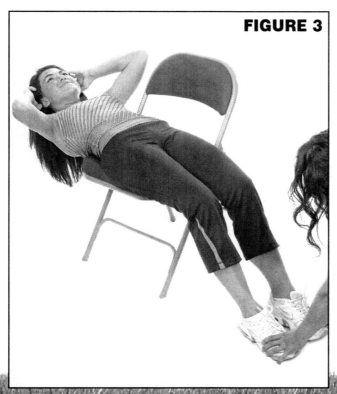

FIGURE 3

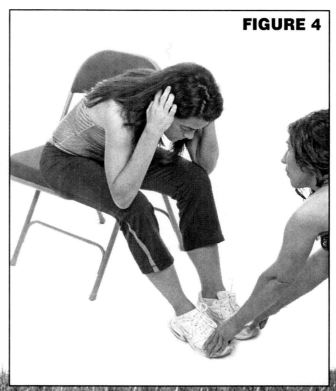

FIGURE 4

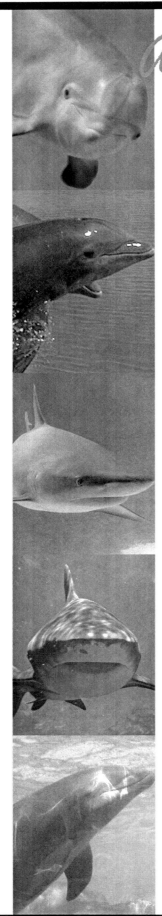

Abdominal Exercises

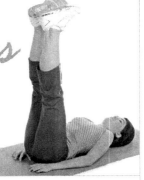

DOLPHIN FLEX I

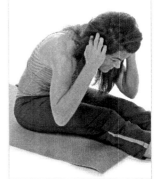

DOLPHIN FLEX II

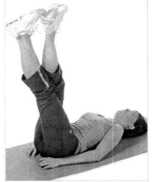

SHARK FLEX I

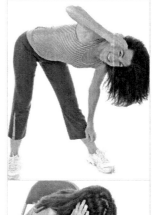

SHARK FLEX II

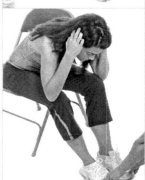

DOLPHIN FLEX III

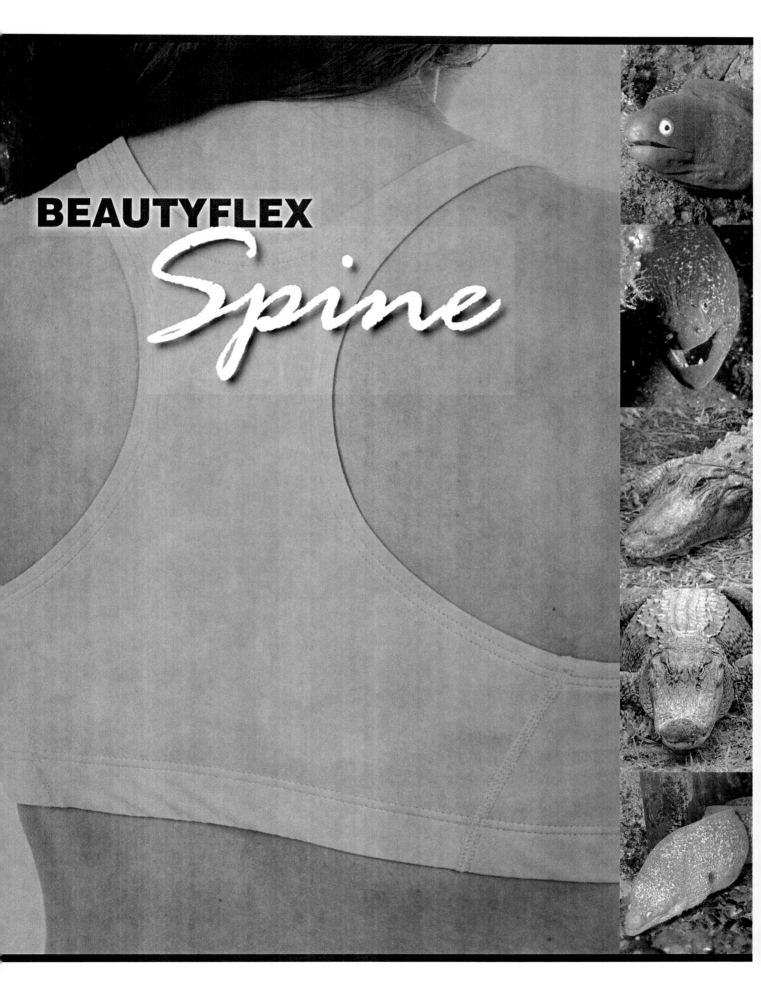

BEAUTYFLEX *Spine*

SPINE WORKOUT

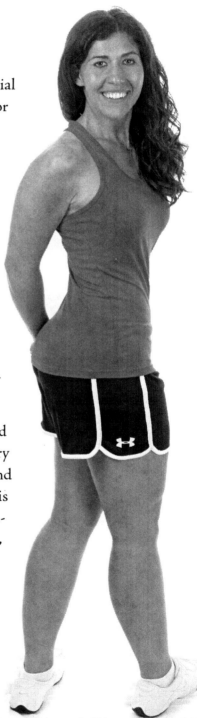

*Y*ou can have a healthy, flexible, energetic spine without the use of special equipment, pulleys, or machines. Just do these five BeautyFlexes for 20 minutes a day.

Wild Workout® for a Healthy, Flexible, Energetic Spine

Like a transformer tower that holds up ultra-high power electrical lines, the human spine holds up the spinal cord, which moves electrical energy—the vitality, radiance, and power of health— through the body.

The spinal column is made up of 24 separate bones (or vertebrae) and two fused bones, the sacrum (with five bones) and the coccyx (with four bones). If any of these separate or fused bones is out of place, energy won't move through the body the way it's meant to. If energy becomes blocked, pain and illness often follow.

Any chiropractor will tell you that your health—physical and mental—depends on the health and flexibility of your spine. Yet very few other exercise courses include movements designed to protect and improve the spine's health and flexibility. The five BeautyFlexes in this Workout imitate the movements of the eel and the alligator, two creatures whose incredibly flexible spines allow them to twist, turn, swim, and strike with purpose and power.

IMPORTANT: Do the BeautyFlexes in this workout slowly and smoothly. Don't bend or twist any farther than is comfortable for you. These BeautyFlexes aren't as difficult as other ones you've done, but doing them will make all the other BeautyFlexes more effective. Now, let's beautify and do the Wild Workout®!

#1—EEL FLEX I

Sit on a chair or stool and fold your arms in front of you. Twist to the left from your waist as far as you can comfortably. Then return to your starting position and twist to your right. Move smoothly and take your time. Twisting to the left once and to the right once counts as one repetition.

LEVEL THREE: 40 reps (20 per side)
LEVEL TWO: 20 repetitions
LEVEL ONE: 10 repetitions

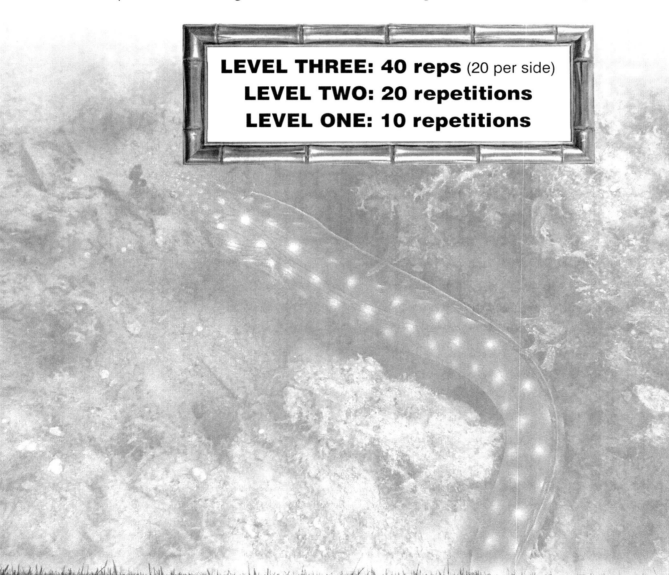

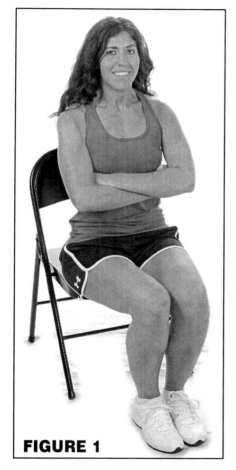

FIGURE 1

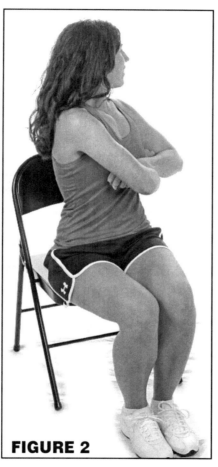

FIGURE 2

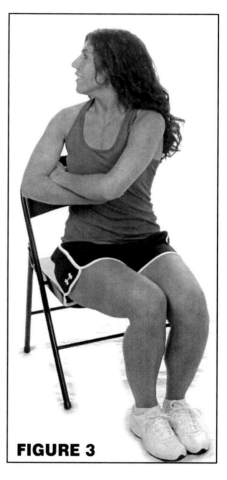

FIGURE 3

#2—EEL FLEX II

*T*his BeautyFlex® is for the upper part of the spine. While these exercises may not seem as strenuous as others, they are critical in keeping a flexible spine.

Sit or stand facing forward and bend your head down as far as you can comfortably. Try to touch your chin to the bottom of your neck. Now, move your head back as far as you can comfortably. Try to touch the back of your head to the back of your neck. Again, move smoothly. Bending forward once and back once counts as one repetition.

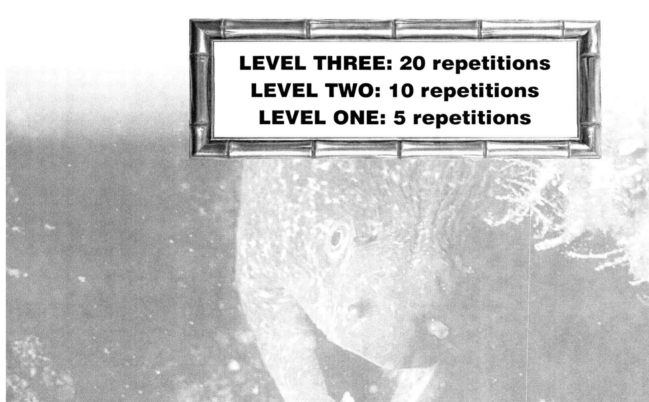

LEVEL THREE: 20 repetitions
LEVEL TWO: 10 repetitions
LEVEL ONE: 5 repetitions

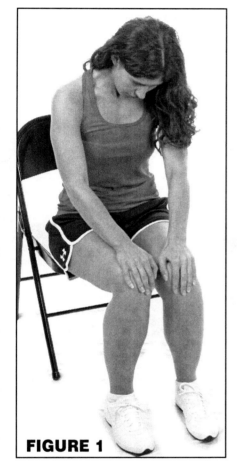

FIGURE 1

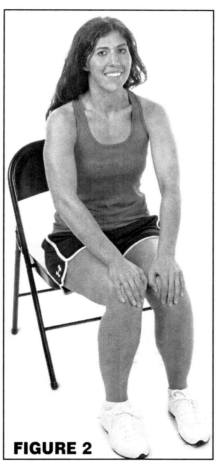

FIGURE 2

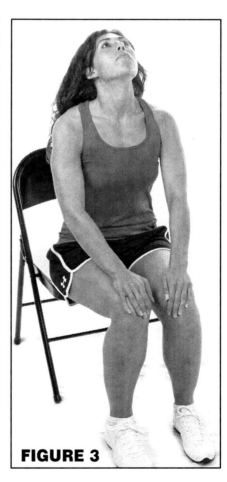

FIGURE 3

#3—ALLIGATOR FLEX I

*T*he alligator is one of Mother Nature's greatest wrestlers, and its best move is the Alligator Roll. Thanks to its flexible spine, it can pull victims toward it by rolling its body. If you don't want to become a victim of back pain, be sure to do this BeautyFlex®!

Stand with your feet shoulder-width apart. Clasp your hands behind your back and twist to your right as far as you can comfortably. Then repeat the movement while twisting to your left. Twisting to your right once and to your left once counts as one repetition.

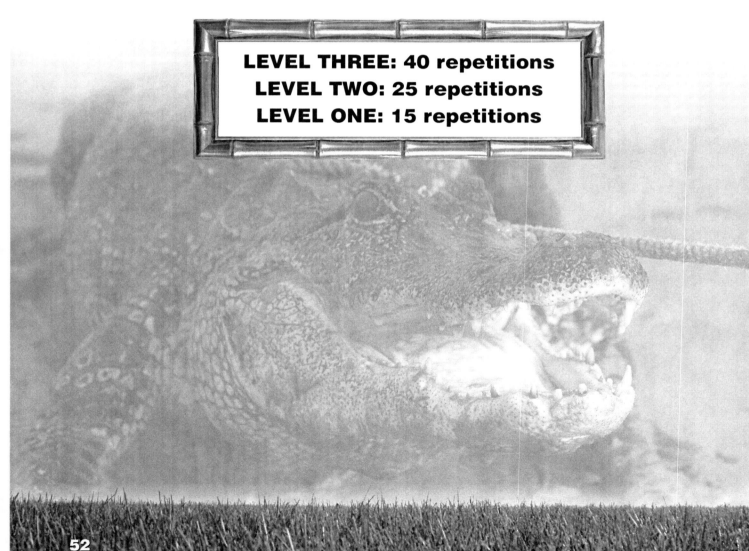

LEVEL THREE: 40 repetitions
LEVEL TWO: 25 repetitions
LEVEL ONE: 15 repetitions

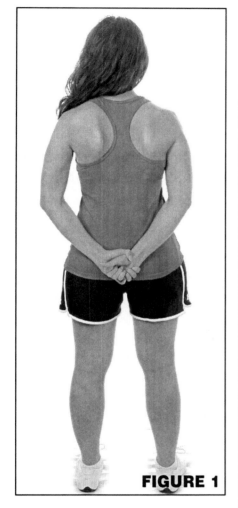

FIGURE 1

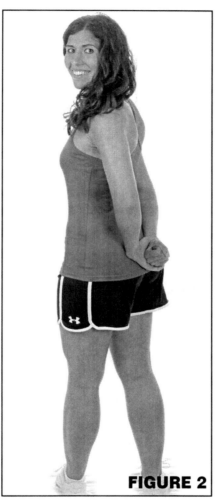

FIGURE 2

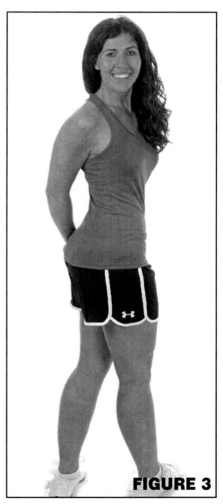

FIGURE 3

#4—ALLIGATOR FLEX II

This BeautyFlex® stretches your spine in two ways, with a forward bend and a backward bend. This combination stimulates the movement of energy—and health—through the spine and throughout the body.

Stand with your feet together and your knees straight. Lift your arms overhead, then bend forward as far as you can comfortably while keeping your knees straight. Stand up again smoothly, raising your hands overhead again and bending backward. Don't try to bend backward farther than is comfortable for you.

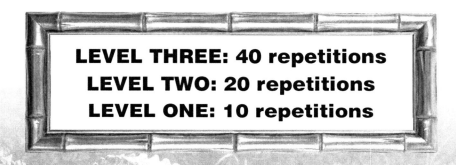

LEVEL THREE: 40 repetitions
LEVEL TWO: 20 repetitions
LEVEL ONE: 10 repetitions

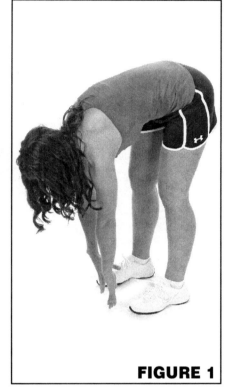

FIGURE 1

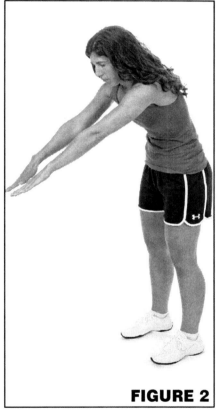

FIGURE 2

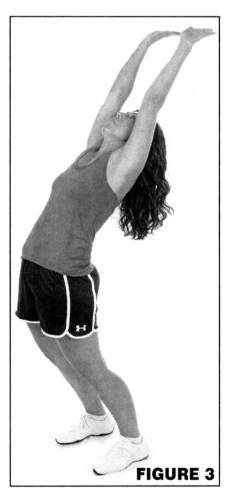

FIGURE 3

#5—EEL FLEX III

*T*he last BeautyFlex® in this workout is one more side-to-side twist. If you've noticed, the eel has no hands, arms, feet, or legs. It keeps fit and full of energy by twisting, turning, flexing, swimming, and striking—all with its body trunk. I am working your spine the same way.

Stand with your feet together, your knees straight, and your arms straight overhead. Twist from the waist as far as you can to your left, then twist as far as you can to the right.

LEVEL THREE: 40 repetitions
LEVEL TWO: 20 repetitions
LEVEL ONE: 10 repetitions

There you are, friend. Practicing these BeautyFlexes consistently and patiently will go a long way toward protecting and improving your spine's health. Always remember that your mental and physical health depend on the health and flexibility of your spine. After all, if you want to show "backbone," you'd better have a healthy one!

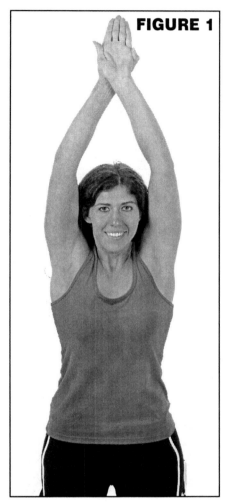

FIGURE 1

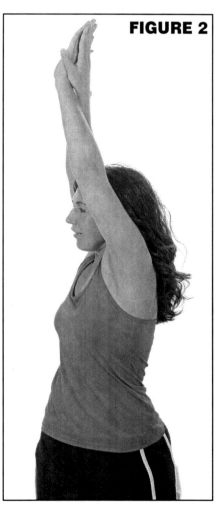

FIGURE 2

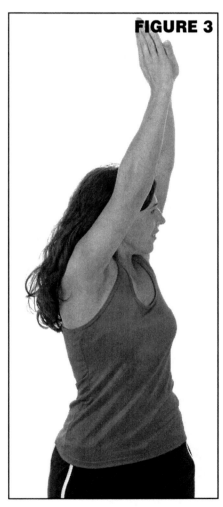

FIGURE 3

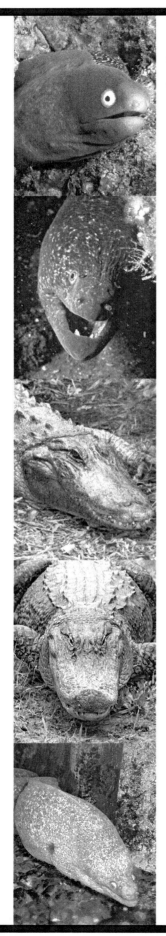

Spine Exercises

EEL FLEX I

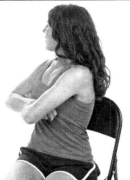

EEL FLEX II

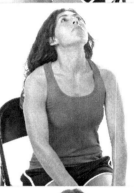

ALLIGATOR FLEX I

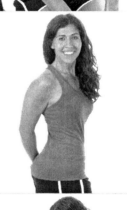

ALLIGATOR FLEX II

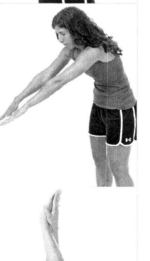

EEL FLEX III

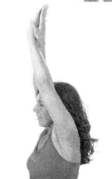

BEAUTYFLEX
Neck

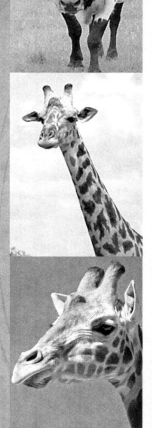

NECK WORKOUT

*Y*ou can have a firm, sleek, sturdy neck with no special equipment, or pills. Just do five Beauty-Flexes for 20 minutes a day.

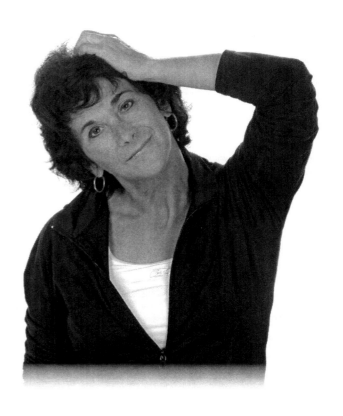

Wild Workout® for a Firm and Sleek Neck

Many women suffer from headaches. Most headaches come from the base of head where it meets the neck. Strengthening those muscles for head and neck health is very beneficial regarding headaches as well as preventing injuries.

Whether you're a woman carrying loads of books and bags, getting pulled at from all directions by children, or you just share the road with tailgating drivers, the BeautyFlexes in this workout can help you build a strong, sleek neck that's both injury-resistant and attractive.

These BeautyFlexes imitate the movements of the bull and the giraffe, two animals whose necks are perfectly adapted to their needs. Thanks to its neck, the bull can use its horns to gore, ram, or toss anything in its path—including bullfighters and 200-pound rodeo riders. The giraffe's long, neck allows it to pick fruit off of tall tree branches other animals can't reach, and to look graceful and elegant doing it.

IMPORTANT: for four of the five BeautyFlexes here, you'll use one of your hands to provide resistance. To avoid injury and sore muscles as you get started, keep the resistance light. Never force your neck. Now, let's Beauty FLEX!

#1—BULL FLEX I

This BeautyFlex® works the muscles toward the front of the neck. Sit or stand, facing forward. Bend your head back as far as you can without straining. Place the palm of either hand on your forehead. Slowly and smoothly straighten your neck as you resist with your hand.

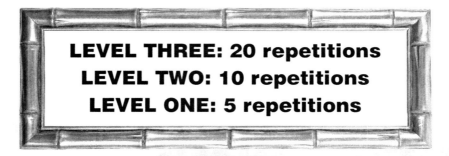

LEVEL THREE: 20 repetitions
LEVEL TWO: 10 repetitions
LEVEL ONE: 5 repetitions

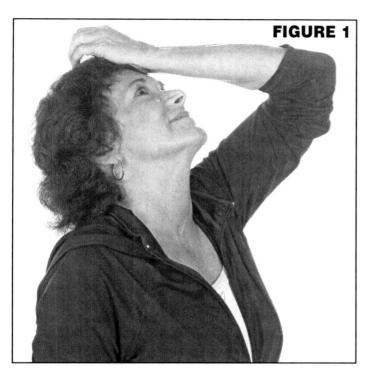

FIGURE 1

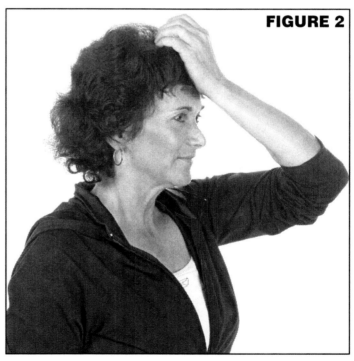

FIGURE 2

#2—BULL FLEX II

*T*his BeautyFlex® works the muscles toward the back of the neck. Sit or stand, facing forward. Bow your head forward as far as you can without straining. Place the palm of either hand against the back of your head. Slowly and smoothly straighten your neck as you resist with your hand.

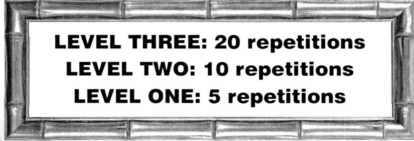

LEVEL THREE: 20 repetitions
LEVEL TWO: 10 repetitions
LEVEL ONE: 5 repetitions

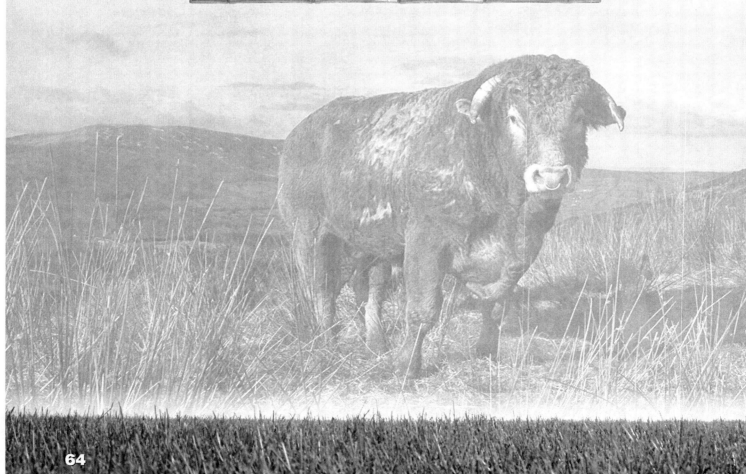

FIGURE 1

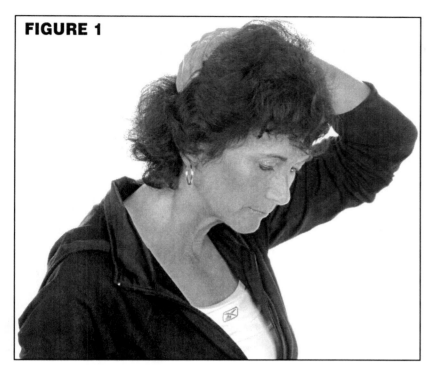

FIGURE 2

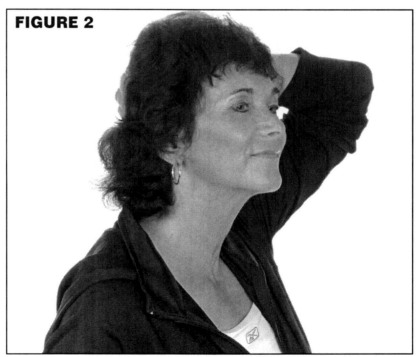

#3—BULL FLEX III

*T*he next two BeautyFlexes work the muscles along the sides of the neck. If you want to build a neck that's strong and supportive, it's very important to work your neck through its complete range of motion.

Sit or stand, facing forward. Bow your head down and to the right as far as you can without straining. Place the palm of your left hand on the left side of your head, just above the ear. Slowly and smoothly straighten your neck as you resist. Then reverse the movement, bowing your head down and left and resisting with your right hand as you straighten your neck again.

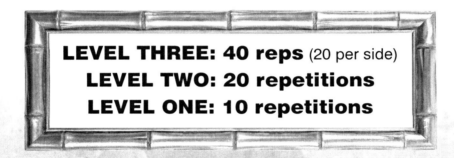

LEVEL THREE: 40 reps (20 per side)
LEVEL TWO: 20 repetitions
LEVEL ONE: 10 repetitions

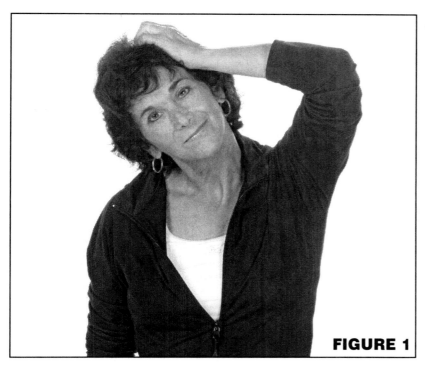

FIGURE 1

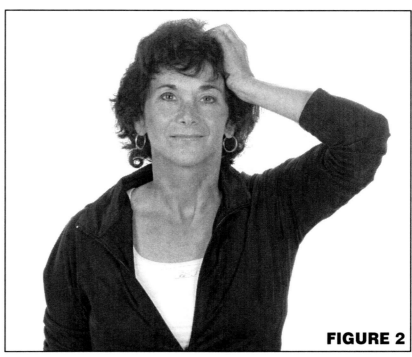

FIGURE 2

#4—GIRAFFE FLEX I

*S*it or stand, facing forward. Keeping your neck straight, turn your head to the left. Place your right palm on the right side of your forehead. Slowly and smoothly turn your head, resisting with your right hand, until you're facing forward again. Switch hands and reverse the movement.

LEVEL THREE: 40 reps (20 per side)
LEVEL TWO: 20 repetitions
LEVEL ONE: 10 repetitions

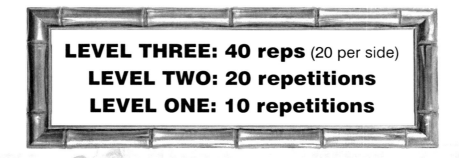

FIGURE 1

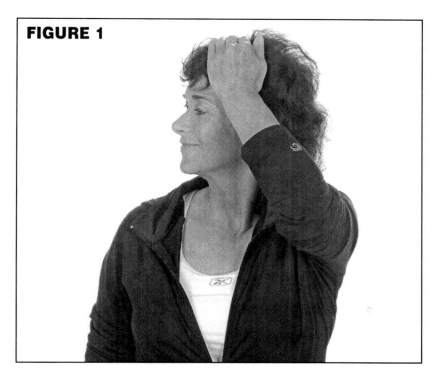

FIGURE 2

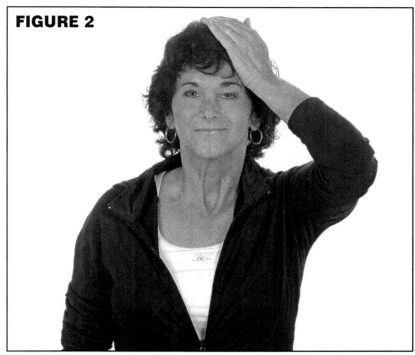

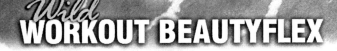
#5—GIRAFFE FLEX II

*T*his BeautyFlex® will give your neck a good stretch as you complete the workout. Sit or stand, facing forward. Bow your head to the right as far as you can without straining. Slowly roll your head, rotating your neck in clockwise circles. Reverse the movement and repeat, rotating your neck counter-clockwise.

LEVEL THREE: 20 reps (10 each way)
LEVEL TWO: 15 repetitions
LEVEL ONE: 10 repetitions

There you go: five BeautyFlexes to help you build a strong, well-muscled, attractive neck. These BeautyFlexes are not hard to do. But if you do them consistently and patiently, you'll help protect your neck from injury.

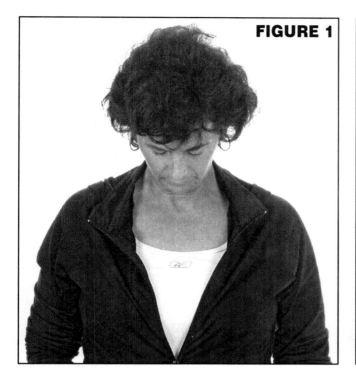

FIGURE 1

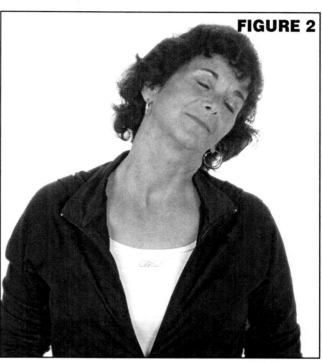

FIGURE 2

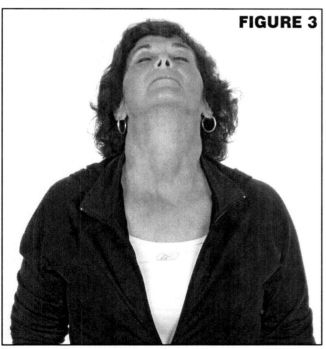

FIGURE 3

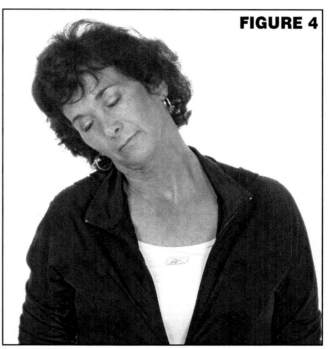

FIGURE 4

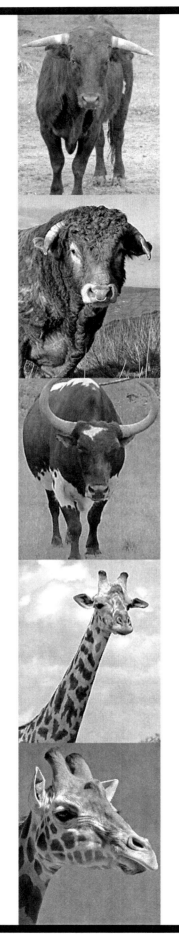

Neck Exercises

BULL FLEX I

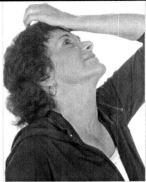

BULL FLEX II

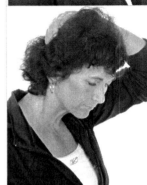

BULL FLEX III

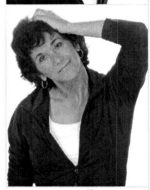

GIRAFFE FLEX I

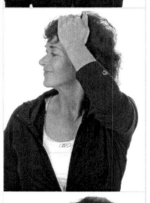

GIRAFFE FLEX II

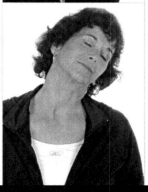

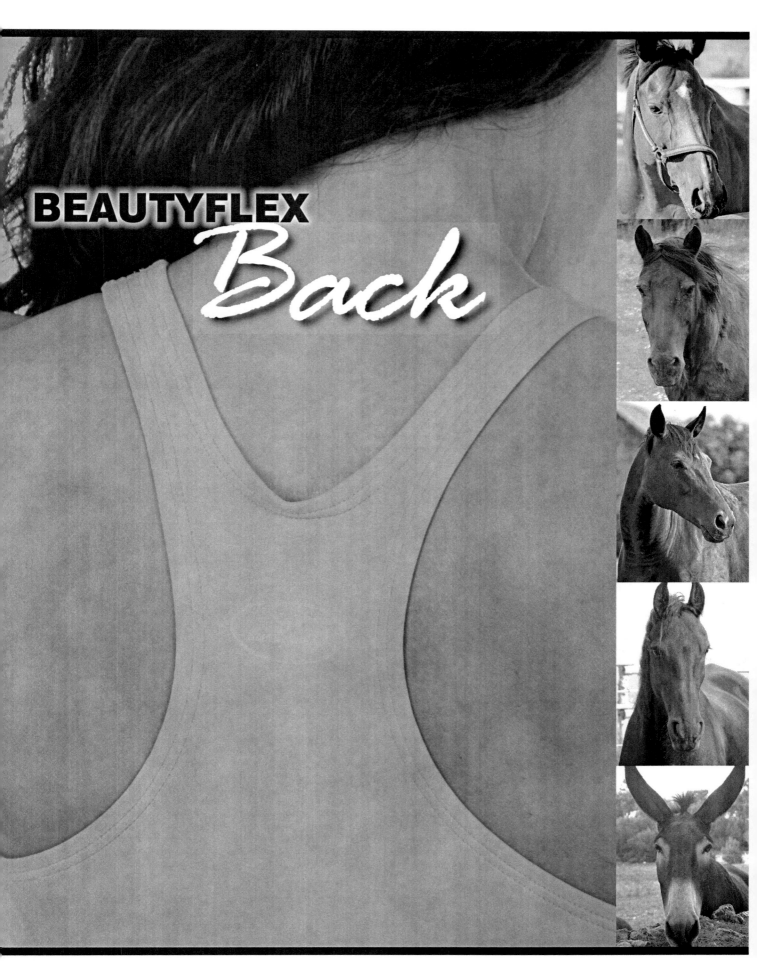

BEAUTYFLEX Back

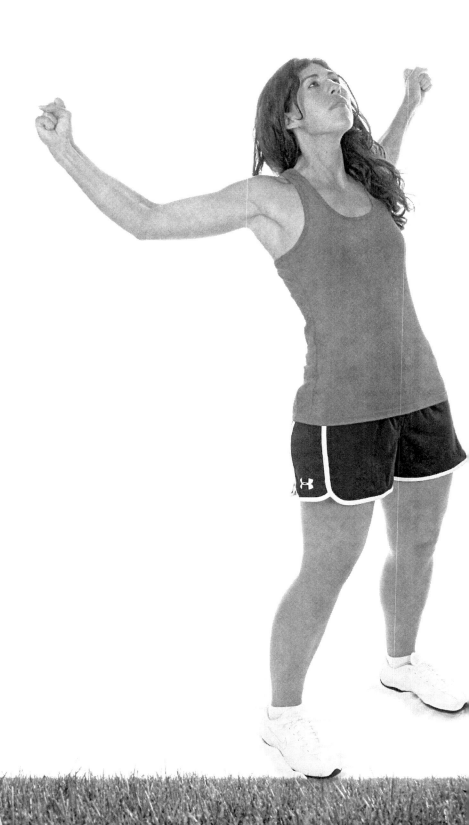

BACK WORKOUT

*Y*ou can have a defined, attractive, strong back without using equipment, weights, pulleys, or machines. Just do five BeautyFlexes for 20 minutes a day.

Wild Workout® for a Well-Defined Back

For thousands of years, one of the hallmarks of a fit, woman has been a V-shaped upper body—the striking effect created by well-developed chest and back tapering down to a lean, stomach. This look fascinated ancient Greek and Roman sculptors, as well. Not all women are created in this fashion however! We as women have different shapes ranging from the tube shape, to the hourglass figure. By flexing our beauty we can be happy with the shape we were blessed with, and enhance our shape to attain the best physique for our figure.

In the animal kingdom, no creature has been more celebrated by artists than the horse for its awe-inspiring combination of speed, power, endurance, and graceful muscularity. Civilization itself has been built on the horse's broad, sinewy back as it has carried riders and pulled carriages, chariots, wagons, and plows. Few people own horses these days, but the engines in our cars and trucks are still rated according to their horsepower.

The BeautyFlexes in this workout imitate the movements of the horse and its diesel-powered cousin, the mule. Practicing these BeautyFlexes with consistency, determination, and patience will give your back new strength to bear your burdens, whatever they are—and without burdening you with the crippling injuries barbells, dumbbells, and weight machines can cause.

Ready? Let's BeautyFlex®!

#1—HORSE FLEX I

*T*his BeautyFlex® simulates the way horses' back muscles work as they pull heavy loads. It will help you improve your balance, too.

Stand with your feet shoulder-width apart. Lean over and interlock your fingers behind your left knee, just above where it bends. Stand up slowly and smoothly, resisting with your left leg as you lift it. Do an equal number of repetitions as you resist with your right leg.

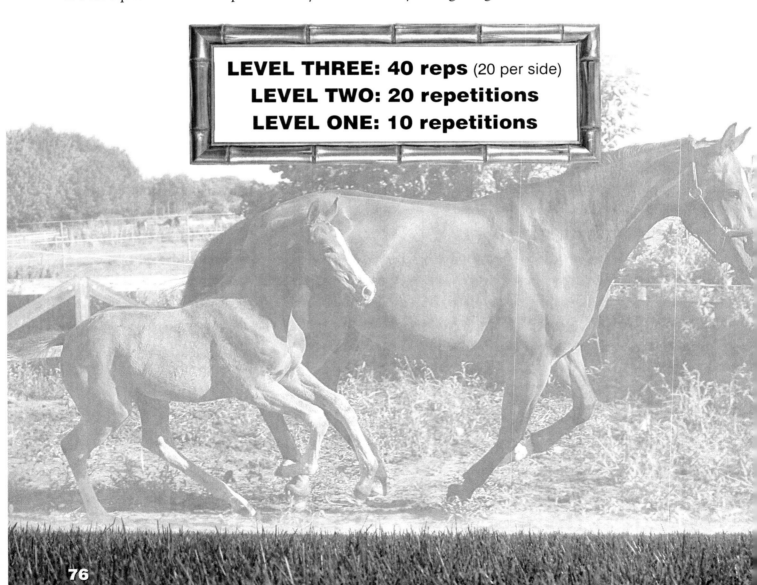

LEVEL THREE: 40 reps (20 per side)
LEVEL TWO: 20 repetitions
LEVEL ONE: 10 repetitions

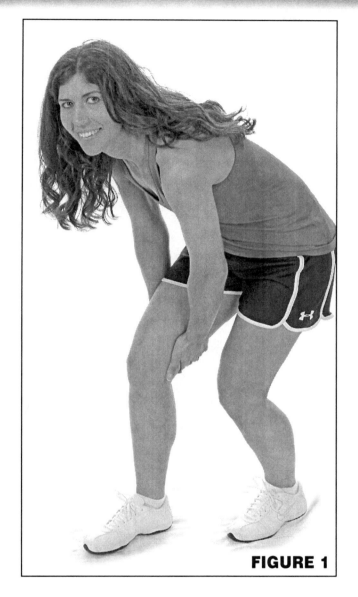

FIGURE 1

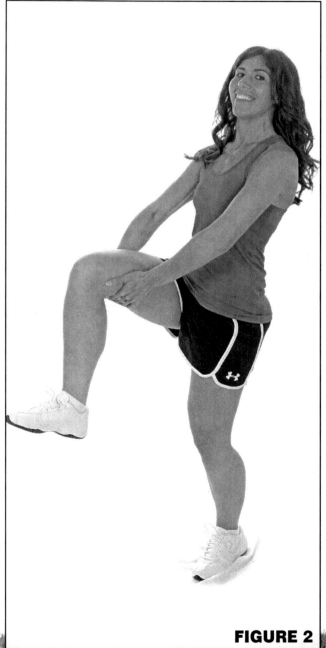

FIGURE 2

#2—HORSE FLEX II

To many fans, bucking bronco horses are the stars of the rodeo. "Broncs" explode out of the chute, their backs flexing and whipping as their riders hold on for dear life. You might have personal experience with feeling like a bucking bronco on days you spend with small children. Your next BeautyFlex® imitates the bronco's movement, but you won't need a rider.

First, set a sturdy chair or stool a few feet away from a heavy piece of furniture, such as a bed, dresser, or couch (you may be able to use the same setup you used for Dolphin Flex III in the Abdominal Workout). Lay face down across the chair or stool and slide your feet under the bed, dresser, or couch. Place both hands behind your head, one atop the other. Slowly and smoothly, raise your upper body until it is parallel to the floor. Then lower yourself.

LEVEL THREE: 25 repetitions
LEVEL TWO: 15 repetitions
LEVEL ONE: 5 repetitions

It is okay if you cannot raise your upper body very far at first. Do the best you can. With time, your strength and range of motion will increase. Do not give up! This BeautyFlex® is essential for building a strong, healthy, pain-free lower back.

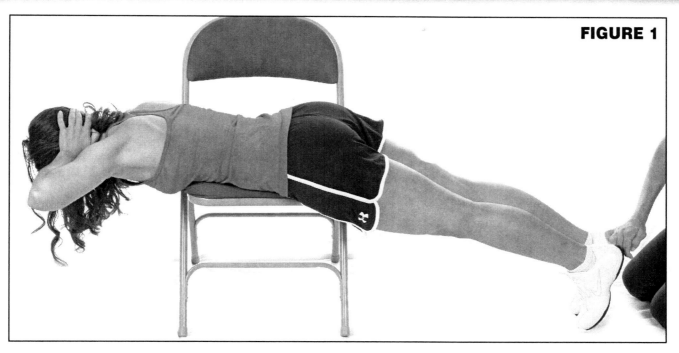

FIGURE 1

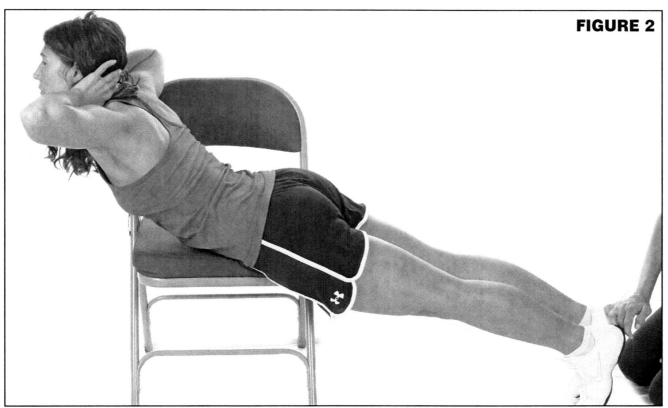

FIGURE 2

#3—HORSE FLEX III

*B*eauty and grace are two qualities women would not mind possessing. Horses are undeniably graceful, whether they are running at the Kentucky Derby or simply brushing flies off their backs by flexing the muscles at the base of their necks. Graceful movements can be observed and learned from God's creatures. This BeautyFlex® imitates that movement and works the upper back muscles.

Stand with your feet shoulder-width apart. Clasp your hands together behind your back at about waist height. Now push your shoulders back and down. Return to the starting position and repeat.

If so desired put a little extra effort into it and your muscles will really stand out. It may seem a little awkward at first, but do them with confidence and the movements will feel very natural after a short time. You will be amazed and pleased by the results—a strong, powerful, muscular back. Envision the goal of how you want to look while you are doing your BeautyFlexes. It will help you put a little something into your workout and help you attain your goal. Keep at it. You can have the body you want. It is attainable. Just don't quit!

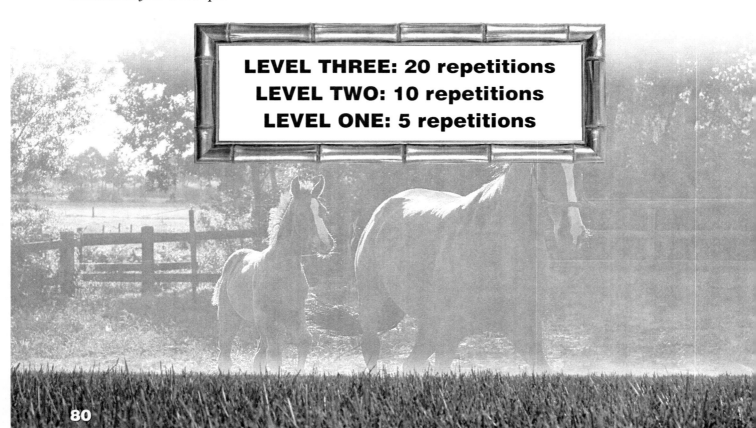

LEVEL THREE: 20 repetitions
LEVEL TWO: 10 repetitions
LEVEL ONE: 5 repetitions

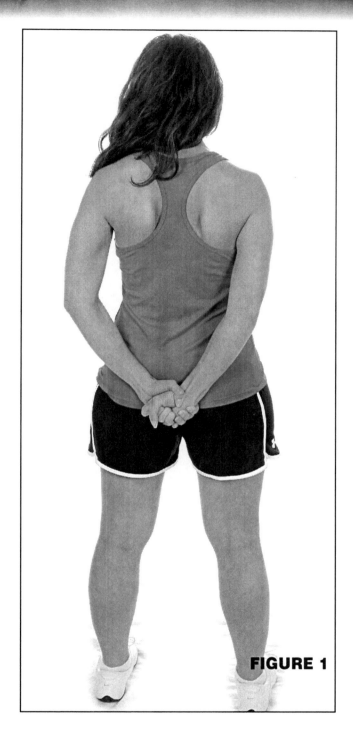

FIGURE 1

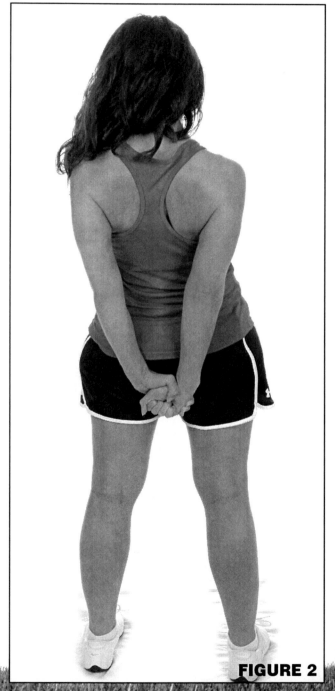

FIGURE 2

#4—HORSE FLEX IV

*Y*ou'll look a little like a lucky horseshoe as you do this BeautyFlex®. Practice it faithfully, however, and you won't need luck to keep your lower back strong and healthy.

Lie face down on a soft carpet or mat. Clasp your hands behind your back. Slowly and smoothly arch your back and, at the same time, raise your legs. Pause for a moment and feel your muscles tense. Lower your torso and legs and repeat.

LEVEL THREE: 15 repetitions
LEVEL TWO: 10 repetitions
LEVEL ONE: 5 repetitions

Like Horse Flex II, this one can be difficult at first. It takes practice to coordinate the movements, but keep at it. Your coordination will improve with your strength.

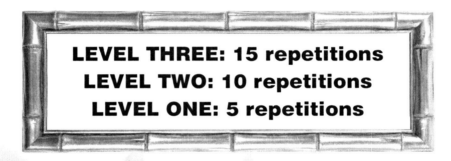

FIGURE 1

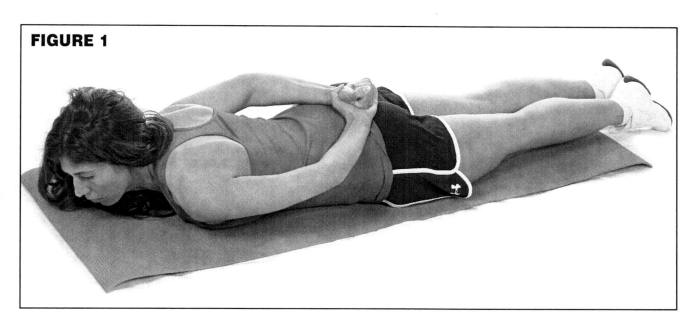

FIGURE 2

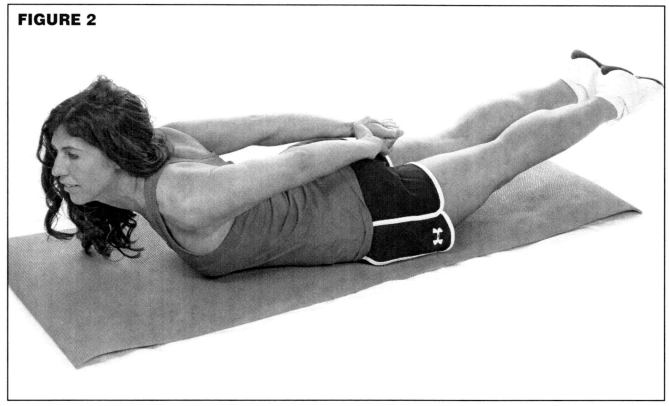

#5—MULE FLEX I

*U*nlike the horse, the mule is not known for its grace but for the raw strength it uses to carry and pull immense loads that would break other creatures' backs. As women we might not want to be referred to as a mule, but we can observe its desirable qualities and express them in a beautiful way. The last BeautyFlex® in this workout imitates the way the mule bends and straightens itself beneath a load.

Stand with your feet shoulder-width apart. Keeping your legs straight, slowly and smoothly bend forward. Touch your toes, if you can do so without straining. Stand up again slowly and smoothly and raise your hands above your head, extending your arms as far as you can to either side. Bend backward slightly. Keeping your arms straight, push them toward each other. Hold this position for a moment, then lower your arms and repeat.

LEVEL THREE: 15 repetitions
LEVEL TWO: 10 repetitions
LEVEL ONE: 5 repetitions

There you go have it, beauty flexes for the back. Practiced with consistency, determination, and patience, these five BeautyFlexes will not only stretch and strengthen every muscle in your back but will teach your body to coordinate and use that strength—something pumping iron will not do. Whatever your burdens, may you stand straight, tall, and determined for as long as you live…with grace, health, and BeautyFlex®!

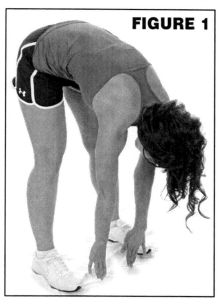

FIGURE 1

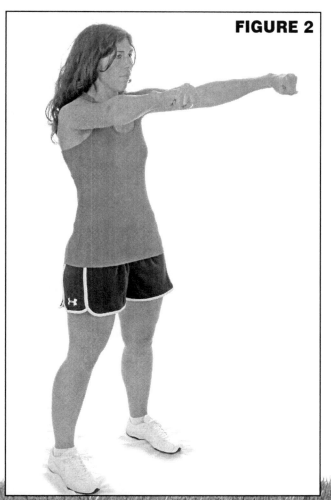

FIGURE 2

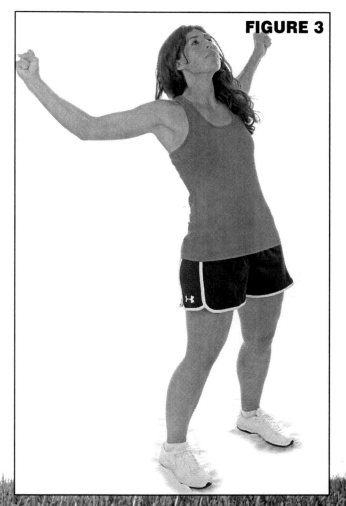

FIGURE 3

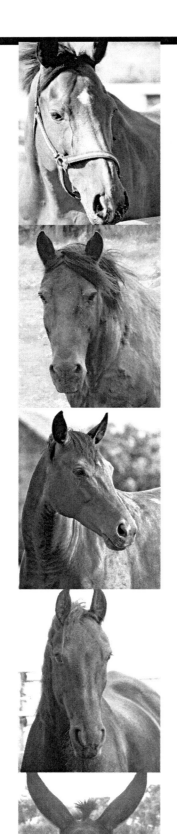

Back Exercises

HORSE FLEX I

HORSE FLEX II

HORSE FLEX III

HORSE FLEX IV

MULE FLEX I

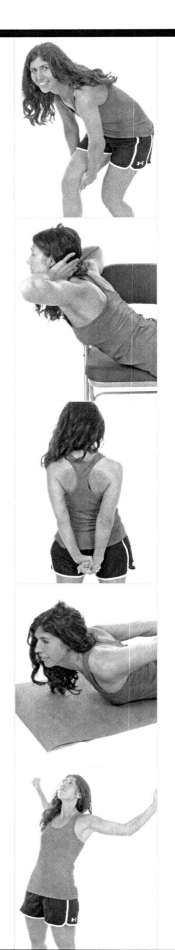

TAKING STOCK

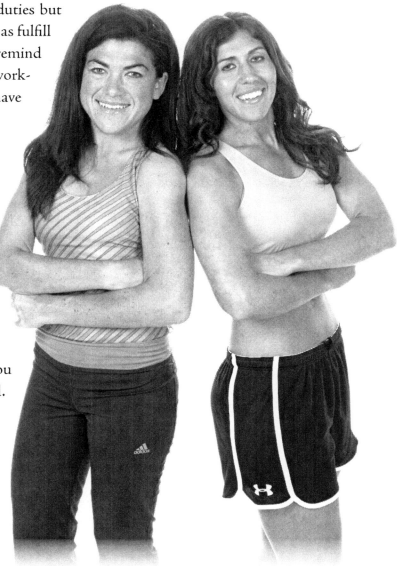

*D*ear Friend, Congratulations! You have made it half way through the course. I am so proud of you. You did not let distractions get in your way such as work, children, school or household duties but you managed to do the Wild Workout® as well as fulfill your commitments! Remind yourself of this, remind yourself how good you felt after completing a work-out session, and remind yourself of where you have come and where you are going. Great work!

If you're following the Workout rotation recommended earlier, you've been practicing the Chest Workout for the last four weeks and have practiced the Abdominal, Spine, Neck, and Back Workouts for a week each. By now, you've begun to reap the rewards of consistent, determined, and patient BeautyFlex®.

Look in the mirror, and be thankful for what you have and the progress you have made. Really, look in the mirror. What do you see? Perhaps you are more defined and toned. Perhaps your troublesome areas are not quite so troublesome. Perhaps your clothes are fitting more loosely. I would like to commend you for your progress and encourage you to not lose your vision of staying fit. You look great. Keep it up!

And how do you feel? Maybe you sleep better. Maybe it is easier to carry bags of groceries, or to weed the garden, mow the lawn, or function in daily duties. Maybe you feel more graceful, more confident in your movements, as you vacuum the living room. At the end of the day, maybe you don not feel as tired.

Well you look great, and this is wonderful, but how do you feel inside. Do you have more confidence to conquer your goals? You are conquering the goal of your body. Now let this accomplishment motivate you to conquer other areas in your life as well. Let the Wild Workout® results be your motivation in other avenues because YOU CAN DO ANYTHING.

Friend, I commend you for your courage. It takes courage to identify changes you want to make, and it takes even more courage to make positive, healthy changes into healthy habits, as you have. I feel blessed that, through Wild Workout®, I have had this opportunity to help you begin to see and feel the body you were always meant to have inside and out.

As you continue this course, be excited for what you have accomplished. As your muscles work, imagine them as you want them to look and feel. And be sure that by learning to flex your beauty the best is always yet to come!

Once more, congratulations!

Sincerely,

Julia Forystek

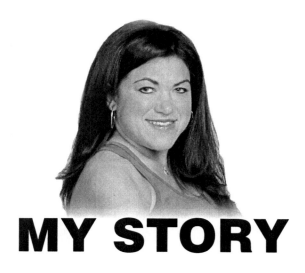

MY STORY

by Julia Forystek

I would like to take this opportunity to share with you exactly why Wild Workout® is so important to me, and perhaps encourage you if you are feeling discouraged. When I was a little girl I had some trials and obstacles. When I was about five years old I started to realize I was not quite normal. My fingers did not fully extend as did most little girls, and my wrists, and other joints were stiff. My parents started noticing as well and took me to several specialists. The more specialists they took me to the more I heard the same answer. "It could be this, but we are not really sure." As I continued to go to elementary school my peers noticed my differences as well, and started poking at me and probing me with questions, such as "what's wrong with you?!" Being a young girl, I simply brushed it off and tried to ignore the questions, one because I wanted to blend in and feel normal, and two because I didn't know what was wrong with me. Each time my parents would bring me to a doctor I would pray "Please Lord let them know what is wrong with me, let them be able to "fix" my hands, and joints."

When my mother brought me to a bone specialist I thought surely he would be able to fix me, and have some answers. He took x-rays, and examined my hands. As he examined the x-rays he said it is simply a tissue-tightness, and there was nothing really wrong with me. He was on the phone while giving me a diagnosis, and quickly brushed my mother and I out of his office. His "important phone call" was a way to mask his lack of knowledge in my matter. I left the office disinherited but had to put a smile on my face anyways. The only comfort I found was the Bible verse my dad and mom taught me very young, "Trust in the Lord with all thine heart and lean not unto thy own understanding, in all thy ways acknowledge him and he shall direct thy paths." (Proverbs 3:5 & 6).

In first grade I had my first tumbling unit in gym class. This is when the children really started noticing my differences, and when I started dreading gym-class. I could not do the cartwheels and handstands as the other children did. I could not even do the simple tumbling moves due to the lack of movement and flexibility I possessed. I wanted desperately to be able to function like the others did in gym class so the children would not laugh at me. I came home from school and sat down on our living room floor about to cry. I looked up at my dad and said, "Daddy, why would God make me like this?"

"Julia" he replied, "Honey, I don't know why God has chosen to Bless you the way he has by giving you hands like that. I don't know why he gave you the ability to use those hands to play the piano so beautifully at such a young age. Or why you can comfort the babies in the nursery, with those hands, the way you do. I don't know why God BLESSED you with hands like that and was so good to you."

His response touched my heart and forever changed my attitude. From that point I realized I could not feel sorry for my self any longer. I could not wish for something I did not have but had to be thankful for what I did have. I memorized the Bible verse, I Thessalonians 5:18 "In everything give thanks, for this is the will of God in Christ Jesus concerning you." Also it was at this point that my dad started teaching me Wild Workout®. He did not have a prescription drug for me, but gave me exercise as my medicine. He would remind me that if I kept my blood flowing, and my body moving, I could not get any worse.

It would not be until I was 23 that I would find out what was wrong with me. Although no doctor diagnosed it, my own extensive research brought me back to when I was nine months old. I was enjoying a day at the park with my mother, and she decided to take me down the curly slide. While riding down the slide on her lap my leg got stuck to the side of the slide and "snap!" there went my femur bone in my left leg! Broken right in half. This incredible break and traumatic experience affected my immune system and resulted in post-traumatic arthritis, or rheumatoid; thereby stiffening some joints.

The miraculous fact is that exercise was the best possible drug I could have taken for this disorder that progressed as I grew. Exercise actually releases a chemical that helps slow and counteract RA. God was in control the entire time. Little did I know that I would go on to teach fitness classes at my university, and conduct fitness seminars as well, teaching other women how to take care of their body.

"Julia is adamant that the 'Biofeedback' required by the "BeautyFlex®/PowerFlex® Method" of mind muscle connection releases healing hormones that are responsible for the amazing health and fitness she enjoys." States a health forum.

Exercise counteracted whatever it was that was trying to slow me down after I broke my leg. The reason I am so mobile today and move so freely is because I kept my blood flowing and body working through exercise. Today I have women coming up to me and asking me how they can get their body to look like my body. They do not see my flaws! Do you have any idea how this concept completely blows my mind?! God is good! I am privileged to be able to teach women to exercise and Wild Workout® in order to reap their beauty's full potential.

BEAUTYFLEX
Legs

LEGS WORKOUT

*Y*ou can have powerful, strong, attractive, well defined legs without using equipment, weights, pulleys, or machines. Just do five BeautyFlexes for 20 minutes a day.

Wild Workout® for Tireless, Attractive, Explosively Athletic Legs

As you begin the second half of this Wild Workout® course, it's no accident that the next workout is for the legs. Ladies, we are known for having great legs! After all, the legs contain some of the human body's largest, strongest muscles. In fact, having strong, healthy legs is so fundamental to our health and fitness that exercises designed to develop the legs also stimulate muscle development throughout the body.

Horses, lions, panthers, and antelopes all run swiftly, thanks to their strong legs. But the creator of Wild Workout® thinks the most impressive legs in the animal kingdom belong to jumpers: to the frog and the kangaroo. I would agree. Having worked with children I have observed from them that the animal jumping qualities are desired as they play. Frogs possess explosively powerful legs that allow them to jump distances many times their own length and to "frog kick" gracefully through the water when they swim. Kangaroos can jump for miles at high speed to escape their enemies, even while carrying their young in their pouches.

Lets learn from the movements of the frog and the kangaroo to define sculpt and shape our legs to be sexy and sleek, yet powerful!

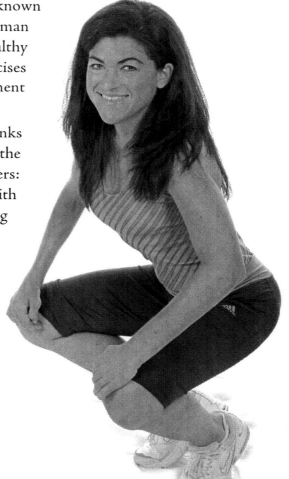

#1—FROG FLEX I

*F*or this BeautyFlex® you'll imitate the frog's position as it springs off the ground—but without becoming airborne yourself. Stand with your heels close together and your toes pointing outward, forming a V. Place your hands on your hips and rise onto the balls of your feet. Keeping your back straight, bend your knees and lower your body as far as you can comfortably. Stay on the balls of your feet. Stand up again slowly and smoothly and repeat.

> **LEVEL THREE: 80 repetitions**
> **LEVEL TWO: 40 repetitions**
> **LEVEL ONE: 20 repetitions**

Balance can be tricky with this one. If you can't keep your hands on your hips and lower yourself without keeling over, it's okay to hold on to the back of a chair as you learn. As your confidence and strength improve, you'll find you won't need the chair. This BeautyFlex® not only works your legs completely but also improves your balance.

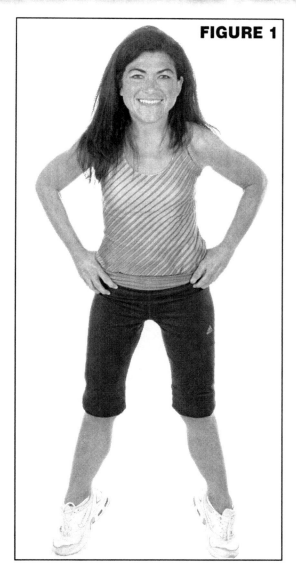

FIGURE 1

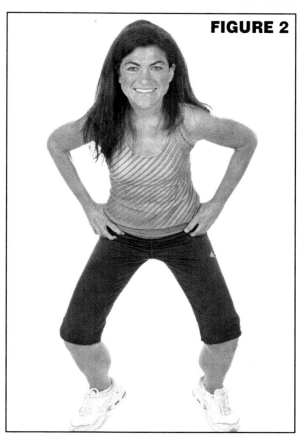

FIGURE 2

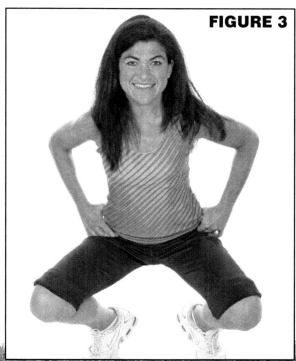

FIGURE 3

#2—FROG FLEX II

*H*ere's a two-part BeautyFlex® for the inner and outer thighs. First, squat down as far as you can comfortably—as though you're playing leapfrog—with your knees spread wide apart. Place the palms of your hands on the inside of your knees. Now try to push your knees together while resisting with your hands. Push and resist for a second or two, then relax and repeat.

For Part Two, squat down with your knees together. Place your palms on the outside of your knees. Try to push your knees apart while resisting with your hands. Push and resist for a second or two, then relax and repeat.

LEVEL THREE: 50 reps (25 per part)
LEVEL TWO: 20 repetitions
LEVEL ONE: 10 repetitions

Be sure to apply enough resistance to make this BeautyFlex® challenging.

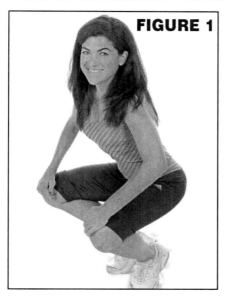

FIGURE 1

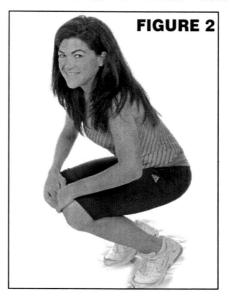

FIGURE 2

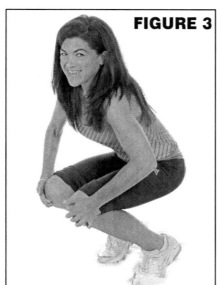

FIGURE 3

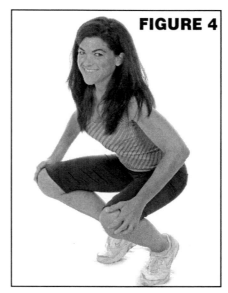

FIGURE 4

Modified

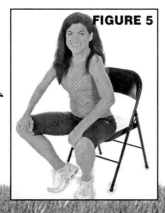

FIGURE 5

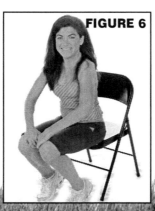

FIGURE 6

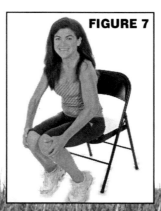

FIGURE 7

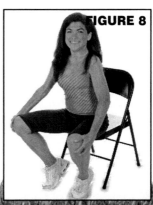

FIGURE 8

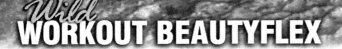

#3—KANGAROO FLEX I

*T*his BeautyFlex® simulates the kangaroo's position as it jumps, as Frog Flex I does the frog's. While standing, cross your legs (like a scissors), distributing your weight evenly on both feet. Hold your arms straight out in front of you. With your back straight, bend your knees and slowly lower your body as far as you can comfortably. Stand up again slowly and smoothly and repeat.

LEVEL THREE: 35 repetitions
LEVEL TWO: 25 repetitions
LEVEL ONE: 10 repetitions

If holding your arms in front of you doesn't help you keep your balance, it's okay to hold on to the back of a chair as you learn this BeautyFlex®.

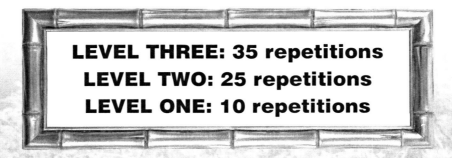

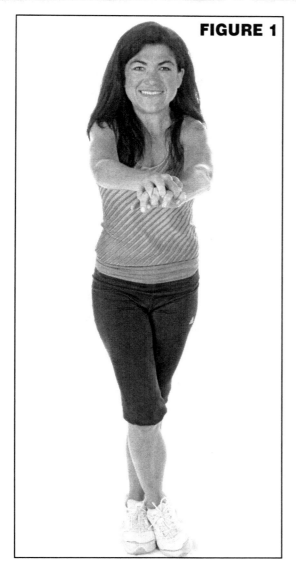

FIGURE 1

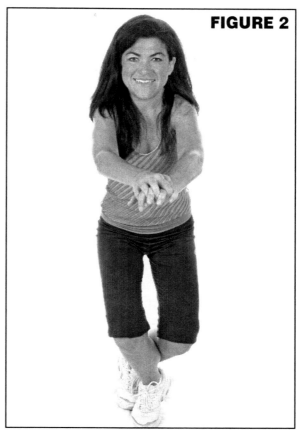

FIGURE 2

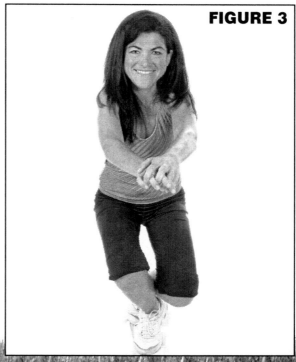

FIGURE 3

#4—FROG FLEX III

*M*ilitaries around the world refer to their scuba divers as "frogmen." Considering such an importance of the frog's movement, we women can take this action into our workout program. This is quite an important observation from these animals. Your next BeautyFlex® simulates the up-and-down movement of the frog's legs as it kicks through the water.

We'll work the right leg first. Stand with your feet shoulder-width apart and your hands on your hips. Without moving your left foot, step back with your right foot. Keep your right leg straight and rest the ball of your right foot on the floor. Bend your left knee slightly. Keeping your right leg straight, push down on the floor with your right foot and lean forward on to your bent left leg. Hold this position for a second or two. Straighten your left leg and repeat. Reverse the movement to work your left leg.

LEVEL THREE: 60 reps (30 per leg)
LEVEL TWO: 30 repetitions
LEVEL ONE: 10 repetitions

FIGURE 1

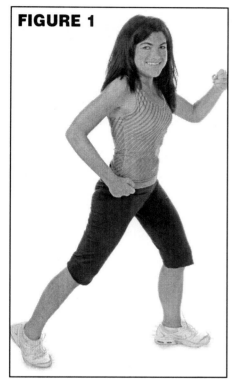

FIGURE 2

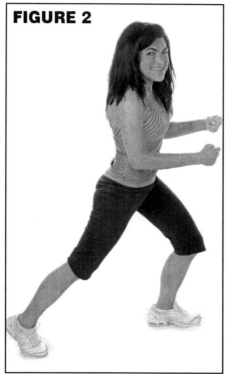

FIGURE 3

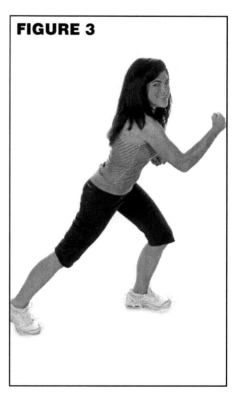

#5—KANGAROO FLEX II

*N*ot only does the kangaroo kick with ferocious power, but also with remarkable flexibility and control—a combination any karate master would envy. This three-part kicking BeautyFlex® will help you develop these qualities.

Part One: stand with your feet shoulder-width apart. Your arms hang at your sides, or you can hang on to a chair for balance. Step backward with your right leg, then kick your right leg forward and as high as you can without straining. Keep you right leg straight as you kick. Repeat the movement, kicking with your left leg.

Part Two: same starting position as in Part One. This time, kick your right leg upward and to the left, swinging it from left to right in a circular motion.

Part Three: same starting position as in Parts One and Two. Now, kick your right leg upward and to the right, swinging it from right to left in a circular motion.

LEVEL THREE: 60 reps (30 per leg)
LEVEL TWO: 40 repetitions
LEVEL ONE: 20 repetitions

Friend, there you have it—a complete Wild Workout® to strengthen, stretch, and shape every muscle in your legs, from your toes to your thighs. With consistency, determination, and patience, you can develop legs that will carry you with confidence, whether you're wearing a tennis outfit, business skirt, or a bathing suit. See yourself achieving your goals, and see how BeautyFlex® helps you achieve them!

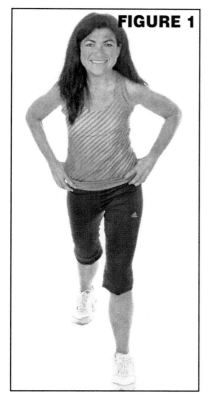

FIGURE 1

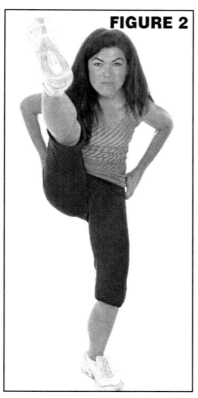

FIGURE 2

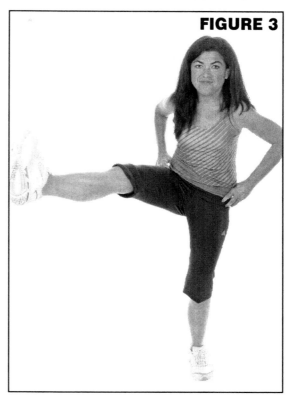

FIGURE 3

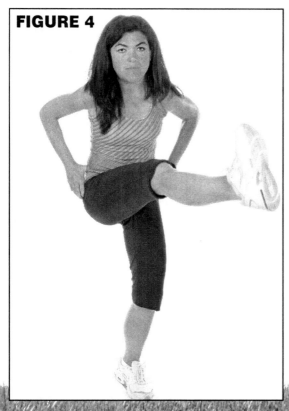

FIGURE 4

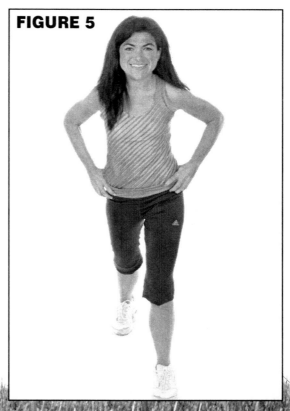

FIGURE 5

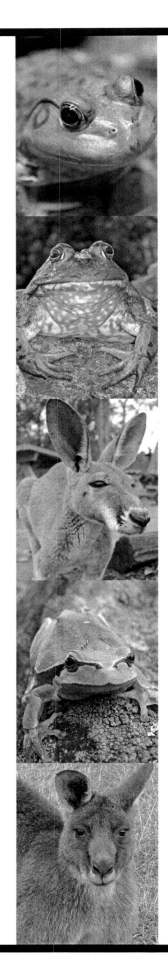

FROG FLEX I

FROG FLEX II

KANGAROO FLEX I

FROG FLEX III

KANGAROO FLEX II

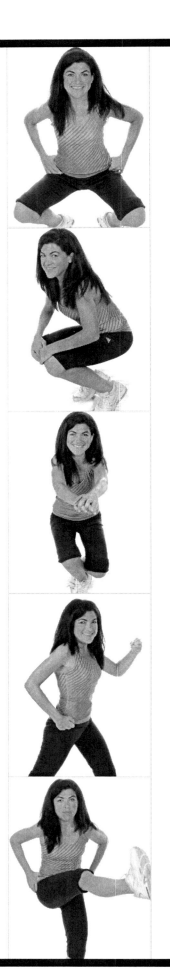

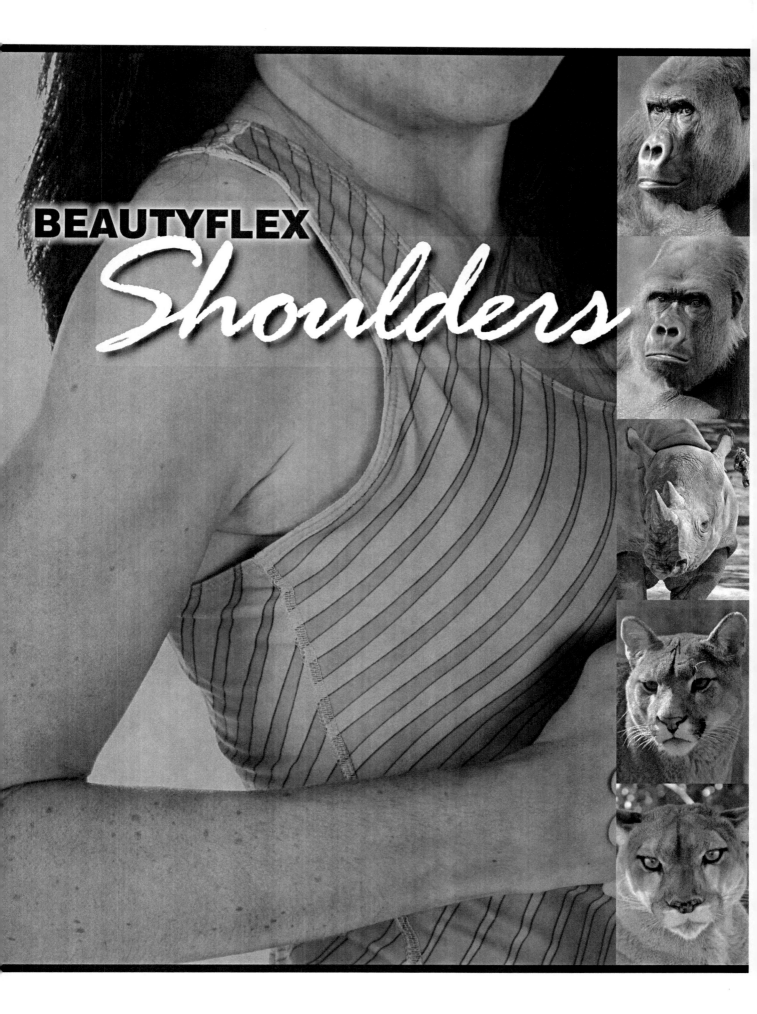

BEAUTYFLEX
Shoulders

SHOULDERS WORKOUT

*Y*ou can have defined, sleek, healthy shoulders without using equipment, weights, pulleys, or machines. Just do five BeautyFlexes for 20 minutes a day.

Wild Workout® for Well-Rounded, Powerful, Healthy Shoulders

It's no accident that when people are feeling burdened, they say they're carrying the weight of the world on their shoulders. We see broad, powerful shoulders and think of heroes—those with the strength to bear heavy burdens confidently and successfully, to protect and nurture others. As women we do not want massive shoulders, but we do want sleek, sexy shoulders that look fantastic in a dress or tank top. I have modified the male's version of Wild Workout® to give results for women that produce that sleek sexy shoulder look.

Bring out that beauty, and get ready to develop and shape sexy shoulders!

#1—GORILLA FLEX II

*T*his BeautyFlex® is similar to a gorilla using its fist to push something away. Sit or stand. Bend your right arm at the elbow until your forearm is parallel to the floor. Make a fist with your right hand and place your left palm over your fist. Slowly and smoothly push your right fist forward while resisting with the left hand. Return to the starting position and repeat. Reverse the movement to work your left shoulder.

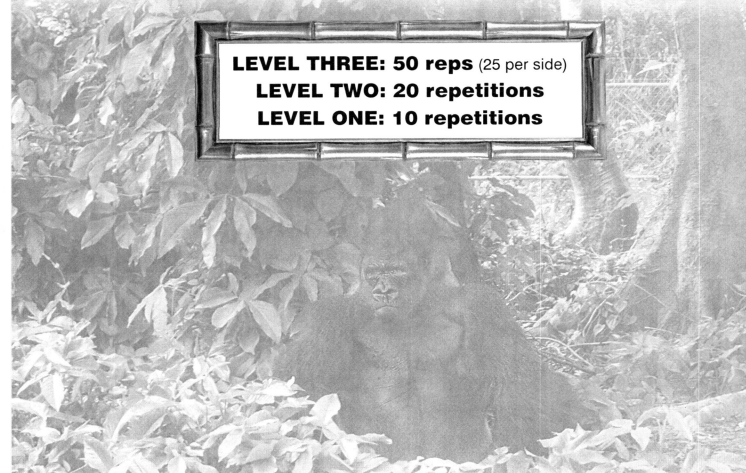

LEVEL THREE: 50 reps (25 per side)
LEVEL TWO: 20 repetitions
LEVEL ONE: 10 repetitions

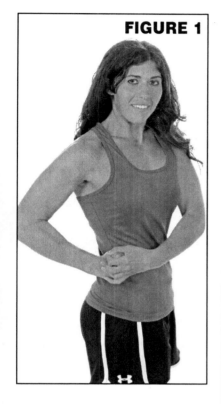

FIGURE 1

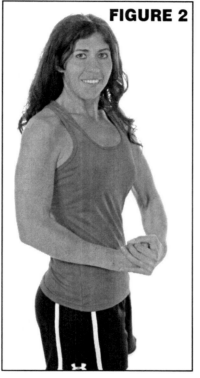

FIGURE 2

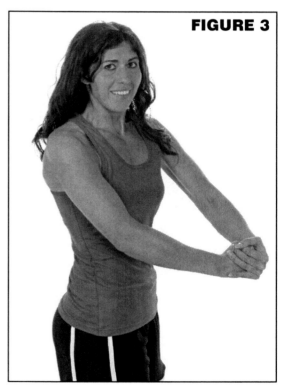

FIGURE 3

#2—GORILLA FLEX III

*T*his BeautyFlex® simulates the way the gorilla pulls itself across and up a tree branch as it climbs. Sit or stand. Raise your left elbow until you're holding it across your chest. Place the palm of your right hand under your left elbow. Slowly and smoothly pull your elbow back down to your left side as you resist with your right hand. Return to the starting position and repeat. Reverse the movement to work your right shoulder.

LEVEL THREE: 50 reps (25 per side)
LEVEL TWO: 24 reps (12 per side)
LEVEL ONE: 16 reps (8 per side)

The muscles of the front, middle, and rear shoulder allow you to move your arms up, down, and around. Developing strong, impressive shoulders means developing all of these muscles. This Beauty-Flex® works the rear shoulder muscles.

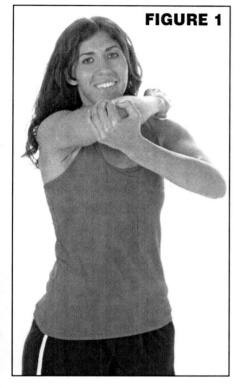

FIGURE 1

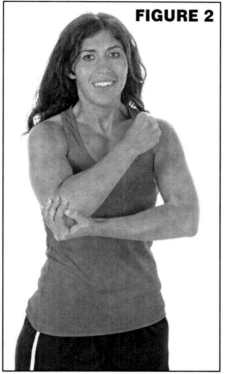

FIGURE 2

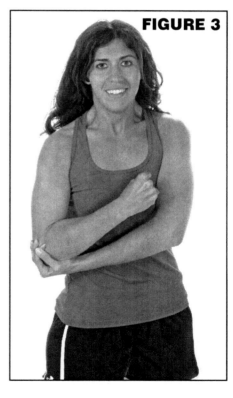

FIGURE 3

#3—RHINO FLEX I

The rhinoceros has huge shoulders! Again we are not going to build muscles that big, so do not worry. We are simply observing their fascinating movements to produce toning in the area. Thanks to the immense muscles along the tops of the rhinoceros shoulders, the rhino can pull its legs through deep, sucking mud. Your next BeautyFlex® simulates that movement.

Sit or stand. With your left hand, reach behind your back and grasp your right wrist. Slowly and smoothly, raise your right shoulder as high as you can, resisting with your left hand. Return to the starting position and repeat. Reverse the movement to work your left shoulder.

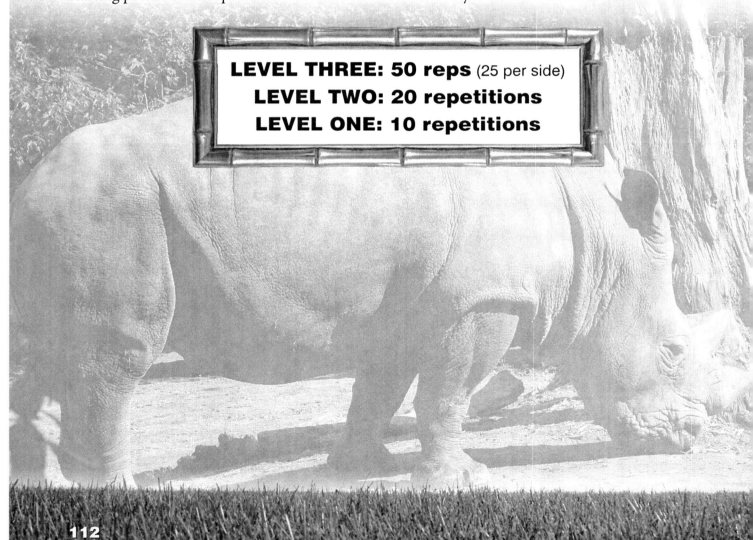

LEVEL THREE: 50 reps (25 per side)
LEVEL TWO: 20 repetitions
LEVEL ONE: 10 repetitions

FIGURE 1

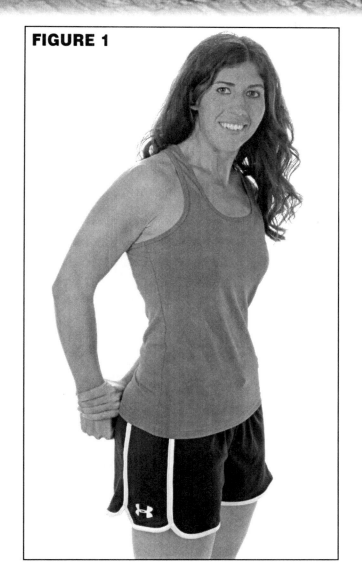

FIGURE 2

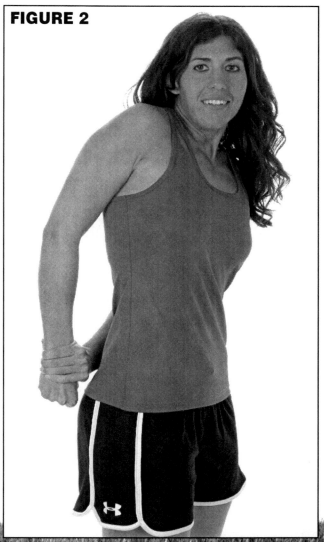

#4—COUGAR FLEX I

This BeautyFlex® simulates the cougar's striking movement. Its developed shoulders allow it to overpower its prey and to wield its sharp claws with pinpoint control. It's excellent for developing the middle shoulder muscles.

Sit or stand. Raise your right arm across your body just beneath chest level. Your right palm should be facing down. With your left hand, grasp your right wrist. Slowly and smoothly push your right arm up and out while resisting with your left hand. Return to the starting position and repeat. Reverse the movement to work your left shoulder.

LEVEL THREE: 60 reps (30 per side)
LEVEL TWO: 20 repetitions
LEVEL ONE: 10 repetitions

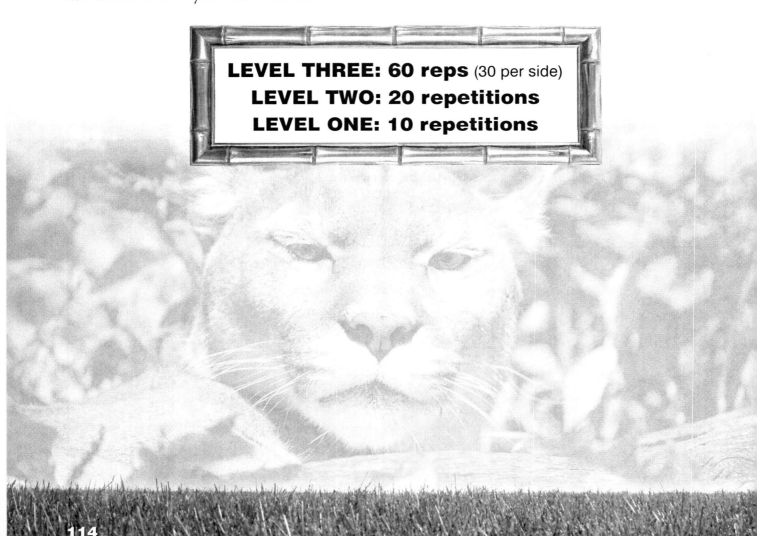

FIGURE 1

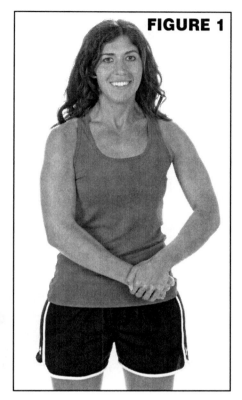

FIGURE 2

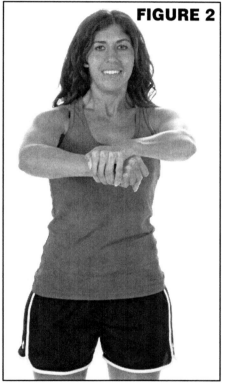

FIGURE 3

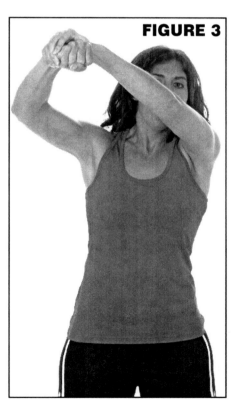

#5—COUGAR FLEX II

*A*fter taking its prey, the mother cougar tears its flesh and begins to feed itself and its young. The last BeautyFlex® of this workout simulates that tearing movement—raw power at its max.

Sit or stand. Raise your left arm across your stomach. Your left palm should be facing up. With your right hand, grasp your left wrist. Slowly and smoothly pull your left hand back toward your left side while resisting with your right hand. Return to the starting position and repeat. Reverse the movement to work your right shoulder.

LEVEL THREE: 50 reps (25 per side)
LEVEL TWO: 20 repetitions
LEVEL ONE: 10 repetitions

Practice these five BeautyFlexes with consistency, determination, and patience, and reap the rewards: shoulders with the strength to defend, nurture, and inspire, and the confidence that goes with them.

FIGURE 1

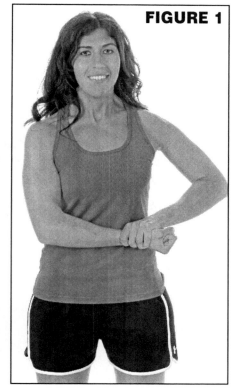

FIGURE 2

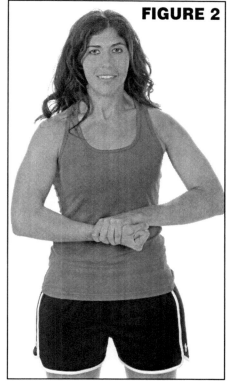

FIGURE 3

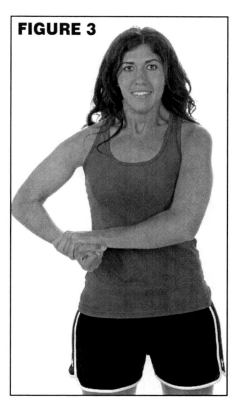

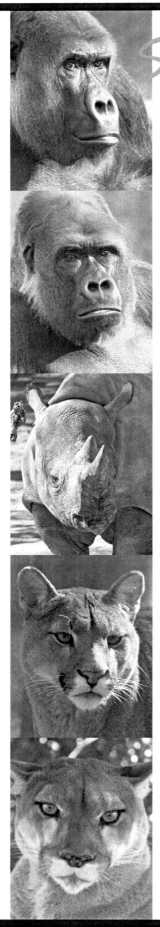

GORILLA FLEX II

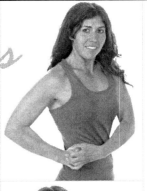

GORILLA FLEX III

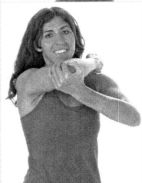

RHINO FLEX I

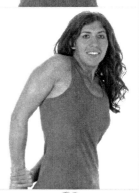

COUGAR FLEX I

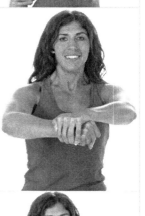

COUGAR FLEX II

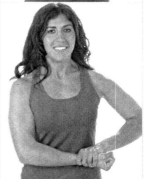

BEAUTYFLEX *Arms*

ARMS WORKOUT

*Y*ou can have strong, sleek, well-shaped, awesome arms without using equipment, weights, pulleys, or machines. Just do five BeautyFlexes for 20 minutes a day.

Wild Workout® for Toned, Shapely, Well-Defined Arms

It goes without question that in order to perform daily functions a woman needs arm muscle. What would you do if you couldn't brush your hair or perhaps hug the one you love? A woman's arm muscles have the privilege of performing many daily functions that often are taken advantage of. With beauty flex we women can keep our arm muscles tight, healthy, and beautiful. We will enable our strength to be enhanced, as well as balanced and perhaps stun a bystander on exactly how strong our womanly arms are.

Wild Workout® for the arms will define to give the arm a sleek sexy definition and rid the arm of the unsightly jiggle every woman dreads! After all, when we stop an arm movement such as waving we want our arm muscles and skin to stop too—not carry on its flapping in the wind!

The BeautyFlexs in this Workout imitate the movements of the gorilla, lion, tiger, and jaguar, five creatures who climb with amazing ease and strike with overwhelming force.

Ready now? Do not get sidetracked. Time to BeautyFlex®!

#1—GORILLA FLEX IV

*T*he gorilla has inspired the creator of Wild Workout® to develop five exercsies in this course. Here is number four. To build impressive arms, it's important to work the biceps, triceps, and forearms from many different angles. This unique BeautyFlex® works the biceps from two angles.

Part One: sit or stand, with your right arm hanging at your side and your right hand palm up. With your left hand, grasp your right wrist. Slowly and smoothly bend your right elbow and pull your right hand toward your shoulder as you resist with your left hand. Lower your right hand and repeat. Reverse the movement to work your left arm.

Part Two: same starting position as Part One. Reach behind your back with your left hand and grasp your right wrist. Slowly and smoothly, bend your right elbow and pull your right hand toward your shoulder as you resist with your left hand. Lower your right hand and repeat. Reverse the movement to work your left arm.

LEVEL THREE: 60 reps (30 per arm)
LEVEL TWO: 40 reps (20 per arm)
LEVEL ONE: 20 reps (10 per arm)

If you have short arms and/or tight shoulders, you may find Part Two difficult to do. Try to let the elbow of the working arm move back and pull your hand toward your armpit as far as you can without straining.

FIGURE 1

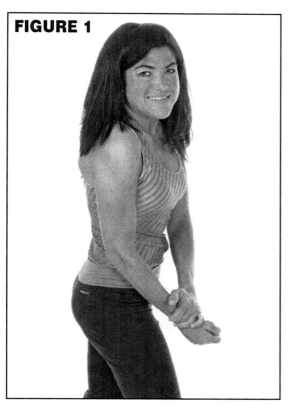

FIGURE 2

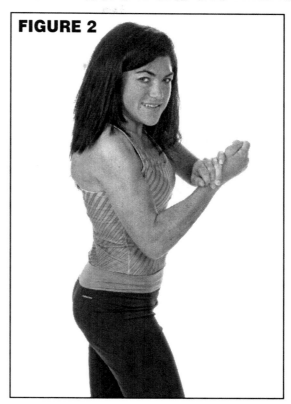

FIGURE 3

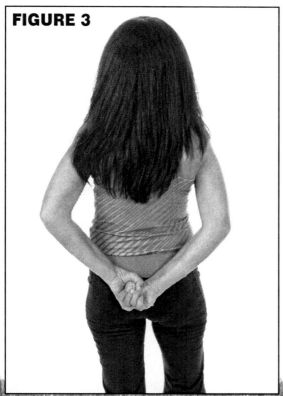

FIGURE 4

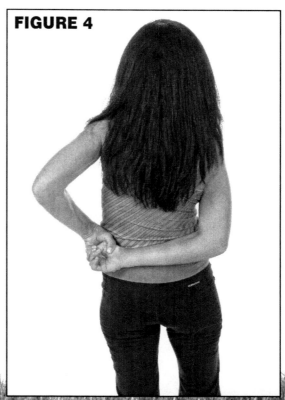

#2—LION FLEX I

*W*hen I was a young girl, one of my favorite pastimes with my dad was to go to the zoo. My favorite exhibit was the lion's den. The male would proudly walk around, while the female would lie in grace, and attend to her young. Their beauty always fascinated me! I would wonder "why are they so defined?" I was amazed at their muscle definition even as a young girl. My favorite time was when the zoo keeper must have put a little too much cat nip into their cage— the lion got a strange zip to his step, and started running around his den.

Wild Workout® pinpoints aspects of the lion noting it's incredible speed and strength which allow it to overcome animals much larger than itself, like the elephant and the water buffalo. Your next Beauty-Flex® (for the triceps) simulates the lion's movement during such expeditions for food and survival.

Sit or stand, with your right arm hanging at your side. Make a fist with your right hand. Bend your right elbow and pull your right hand toward your shoulder. With your left hand, grasp your right fist from beneath. Keeping your right elbow close to your side, slowly and smoothly push your right hand down and out as you resist with your left hand. Raise your right hand and repeat. Reverse the movement to work your left arm.

LEVEL THREE: 50 reps (25 per side)
LEVEL TWO: 30 repetitions
LEVEL ONE: 10 repetitions

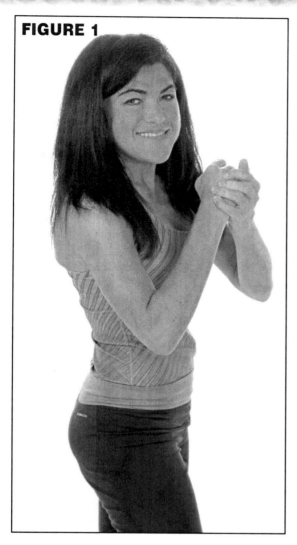

FIGURE 1

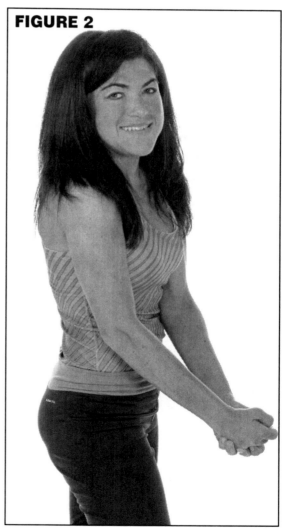

FIGURE 2

#3—TIGER FLEX I

*W*hen women are beautifying their face, and applying make-up to enhance what they were already blessed with, they usually do not put on only one shade of eye shadow, or apply lipstick alone. Each area needs enhancement from each angle. The same concept should be applied when toning your body. Like Lion Flex I, this next BeautyFlex® also works the triceps, but from a different angle.

Sit or stand. Raise your right arm and hold it across your chest. With your left hand, grasp the back of your right wrist. Keeping your right upper arm close to your side, slowly and smoothly push your right forearm up and out while resisting with your left hand. Return to the starting position and repeat. Reverse the movement to work your left arm.

LEVEL THREE: 40 reps (20 per side)
LEVEL TWO: 20 repetitions
LEVEL ONE: 10 repetitions

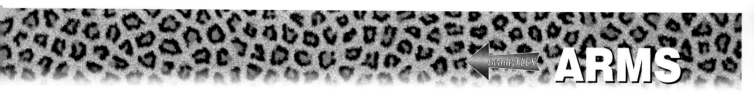
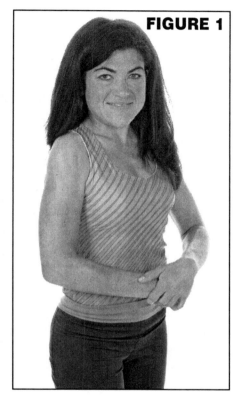

FIGURE 1

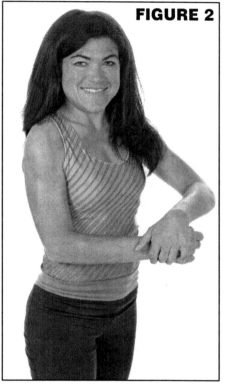

FIGURE 2

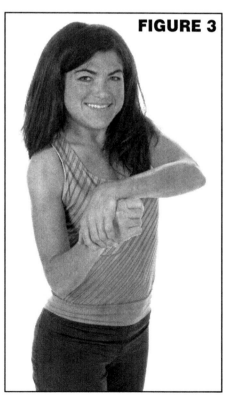

FIGURE 3

#4—JAGUAR FLEX I

*I*t is amazing to watch a slow-motion film of a running jaguar. With every stride, the jaguar pulls itself forward, then stretches its legs, grasps the ground with its feet, and pulls again. This BeautyFlex® simulates these movements and works the biceps, triceps, and forearms all at once.

Sit or stand, with your arms hanging at your sides. With your thumbs facing forward, make your hands into tight fists. Slowly and smoothly, bend both of your arms at the elbows and twist your fists until your palms are facing the tops of your shoulders (like you're a bodybuilder doing a "double biceps" pose). Lower your arms slowly and smoothly. When you return to the starting position, push back on your arms (like you're trying to bend them backward at the elbows) for a second or two. Repeat.

LEVEL THREE: 20 repetitions
LEVEL TWO: 10 repetitions
LEVEL ONE: 5 repetitions

Keep your fists tight and feel the tension in your forearms. As you raise your fists, feel the tension in your biceps. As you lower your fists and push back on your arms, feel the tension in your triceps.

FIGURE 1

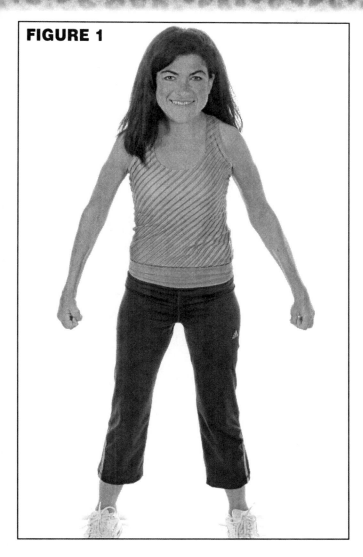

FIGURE 2

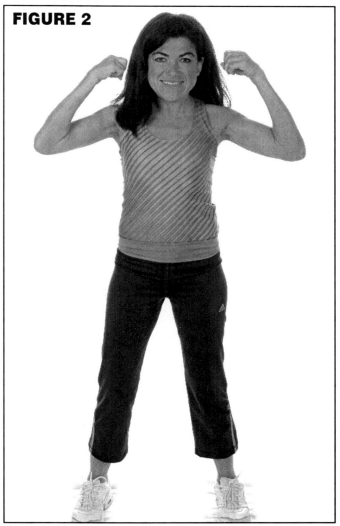

#5—GORILLA FLEX V

*T*his Gorilla Flex is a fine all-in-one BeautyFlex® for your biceps, triceps, and forearms.

Part One: sit or stand, with your arms hanging at your sides. Your hands should be open with the palms facing your sides. Push back on your arms (like you did for Jaguar Flex I) for a second or two. Now shake the tension out of your arms and relax for a few moments.

Part Two: next, make a fist with your right hand. Bend your right arm at the elbow and twist your fist until your palm is facing the top of your right shoulder (as you did with both arms for Jaguar Flex I). Hold this position for a second or two, then relax your right arm.

Part Three: same as for Part Two, but reverse the movement to work your left arm. One cycle through all three parts counts as one repetition.

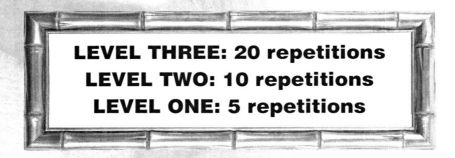

LEVEL THREE: 20 repetitions
LEVEL TWO: 10 repetitions
LEVEL ONE: 5 repetitions

There you have it ladies. A complete way to define and beautify the arms you were blessed with. Thanks to the strong foundation you have built through practicing the previous Workouts, adding these concentrated BeautyFlexes to your routine will quickly produce the results you desire. See and feel your muscles as they work, and imagine them gaining the shape you are seeking. After all, what the mind believes, the body will achieve! You are beautiful. Enhancing your arms allows you to enhance the whole package thus bringing out your inner confidence.

FIGURE 1

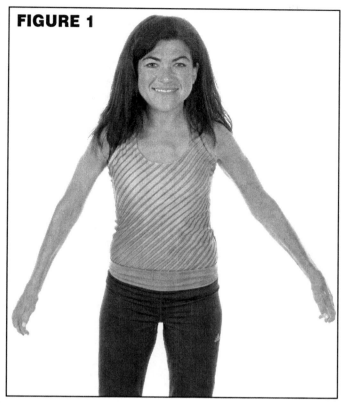

FIGURE 2

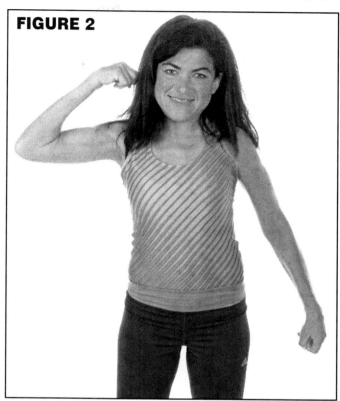

FIGURE 3

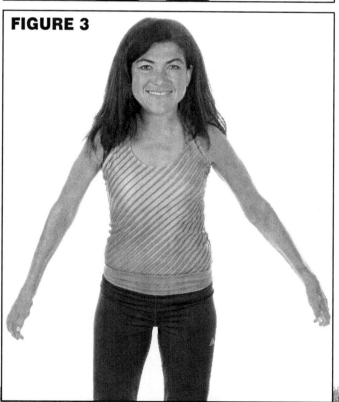

FIGURE 4

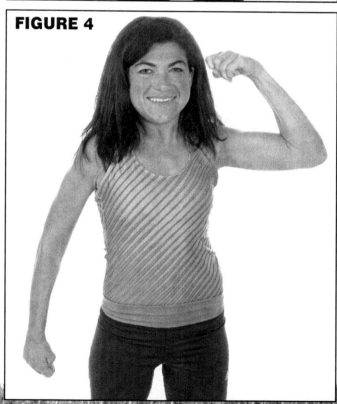

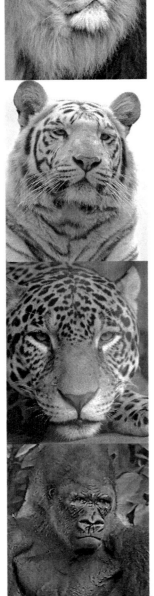

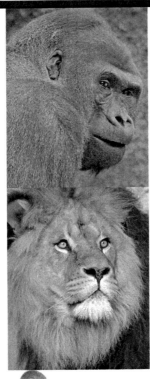

Arm Exercises

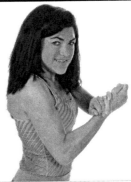

GORILLA FLEX IV

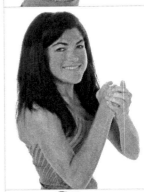

LION FLEX I

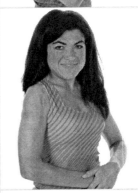

TIGER FLEX I

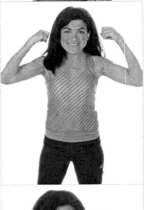

JAGUAR FLEX I

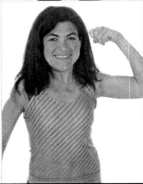

GORILLA FLEX V

BEAUTYFLEX

Speed, Energy & Endurance

SPEED, ENERGY & ENDURANCE WORKOUT

*Y*ou can have speed, energy, and endurance without using equipment, weights, pulleys, or machines. Just do five BeautyFlexes for 20 minutes a day.

Wild Workout® for Speed, Energy, and Endurance

Women today are always on the go. They are running from destination to destination, being super mom, super student, or super employee! Often we end up feeling fatigued and not so super. Women need to take a few tips from animals to keep up our energy and endurance during these typical days. Not only are animals beautiful but as the creator of Wild Workout® emphasizes in his PowerFlex® book, "show" means "go." That is, creatures can actually do everything they look like they can do. The stocky, short-legged mule can actually haul huge loads up and over mountain passes. The lean, sinewy cheetah can actually accelerate to 67 miles per hour in three seconds flat.

If you've practiced the last eight Workouts with consistency, determination, and patience, you've transformed your "show." The Chest Workout helped you lift and define your chest. The Back Workout helped you develop a toned upper body. The Shoulder and Arm Workouts helped you shape your shoulders and arms.

Now, before you graduate, you are ready for a Workout that will work your whole body, all at once. The following Workout begins and ends with a stretch and challenges you to climb, dash, and trot. These activities will teach your body how to coordinate and use the strength and fitness you have already developed and will build your speed, energy, and endurance. It will enable you to conquer each day in record time, all while balancing life and still looking beautiful. Your glow will be radiating from your confidence and energy within. On your mark! Get set (you can do it)! BeautyFlex®!

#1—CHEETAH FLEX I

*I*f you are a woman who has pets, you will know that cats…shred…everything! It doesn't matter whether they are super-predators, such as lions, tigers, or cheetahs, or your cute little housecat who demolishes your elegant sofa! They reach forward with their front paws, grab the grass (or carpet or couch), pull back, and stretch their back and legs. They don't do it to be nasty, but to strengthen their muscles and stay limber. This first BeautyFlex® imitates that movement (without trashing the furniture).

Stand with your feet shoulder-width apart and your hands on your hips. Keeping your legs straight, bend forward slowly and smoothly as far as you can without straining. With your right hand, try to touch the floor in front of your left foot. Return to the starting position, then bend forward again. With your left hand, try to touch the floor in front of your right foot. Return to the starting position and repeat.

LEVEL THREE: 50 reps (25 per side)
LEVEL TWO: 30 repetitions
LEVEL ONE: 20 repetitions

Don't worry if you can't touch the floor at first, or even your ankle. If you do not feel comfortable reaching below your knee simply—start where you are. Never, ever strain! Practice this BeautyFlex® with consistency, determination, and patience, and see how quickly your flexibility and endurance improve.

FIGURE 1

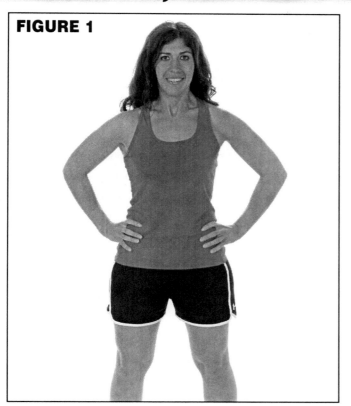

FIGURE 2

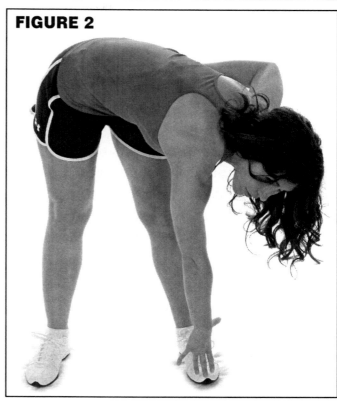

FIGURE 3

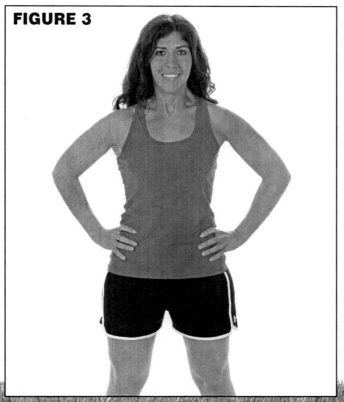

FIGURE 4

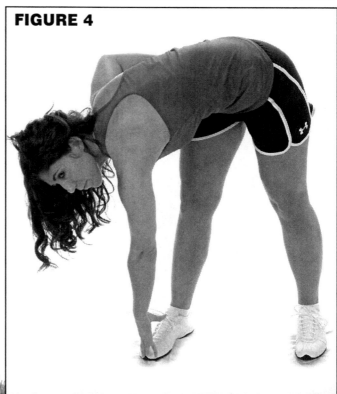

#2—ELK CLIMB

I love to spend days hiking in the mountains. I have seen some of the most breath-taking beautiful views while being high in the Appalachian Mountains or the Blue Ridge Mountains. Thanks to regular BeautyFlex®, I have the strength, energy, and endurance to hike and climb to view such beauty. I feel blessed that I can climb high enough see and appreciate sights people can not see from their cars such as flowing waterfalls, and frolicking animals deep in the meadows.

Fortunately, you do not need a mountain to build the fitness to climb one. Just find some stairs. A set of stadium steps or the stairs at an office or apartment building would be ideal, but you can get the same results climbing the stairs in your home.

Once you have found some stairs, run up and down them if you can, but if that is a strain, it's fine to walk. Do not try to move so fast that you stumble or cannot get your breath. This BeautyFlex® will build your agility and endurance quickly. One trip up and down counts as one repetition.

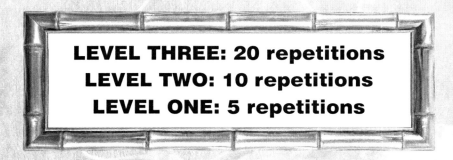

LEVEL THREE: 20 repetitions
LEVEL TWO: 10 repetitions
LEVEL ONE: 5 repetitions

Note: These are general guidelines only. The longer your set of stairs is, the fewer repetitions you'll need.

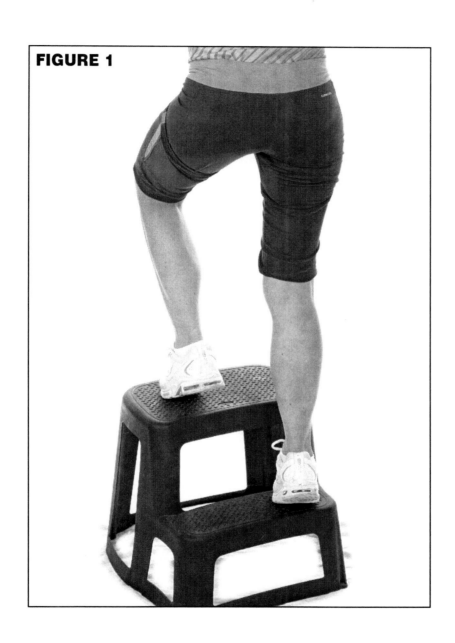

FIGURE 1

#3—CHEETAH DASH

*M*any creatures are celebrated for their speed such as the thoroughbred horse and the greyhound, but the fastest sprinter—hands down—is the cheetah. When chasing its prey, the cheetah can accelerate to highway speed limits more quickly than most cars.

If you are a busy mom, active employee, or assertive student you know that the speed of you accomplishment determines certain success. However if you are an athlete, you know that winning often depends on speed. It's the difference between getting to the ball or losing points, crossing the finish line first or last. The difference between wining the marathon and losing being left in the dust. This BeautyFlex® will enhance and increase your speed. First, pace off and mark a 40-yard stretch of grass (at a park or schoolyard or on your own lawn) or track (at a school athletic field) or pavement (on a lightly-traveled street or sidewalk). Now, sprint the distance. Lift your knees and pump your arms, and don't let up until you've run through your finish line. Rest for 15 seconds (either timed with a stopwatch or counted to yourself), then sprint back to your starting point.

LEVEL THREE: 10 repetitions
LEVEL TWO: 7 repetitions
LEVEL ONE: 5 repetitions

Even if you are not an athlete, practicing this BeautyFlex® can give you a burst of speed to catch a bus or cross a busy street. It can help you look better, too. Research has shown that sprinting not only burns fat more effectively than long distance running but that it builds muscle, too along with burning more calories after your workout is done! If you are new to sprinting, do not run all out at first—you do not want to pull a muscle. Feel free to rest for more than 15 seconds between repetitions, if you need to. In time, you will not need so much rest. Do not strain! If you would rather not sprint, that is okay—fast walking works well too. And you do not need grass, track, or pavement—a large room will do.

FIGURE 1

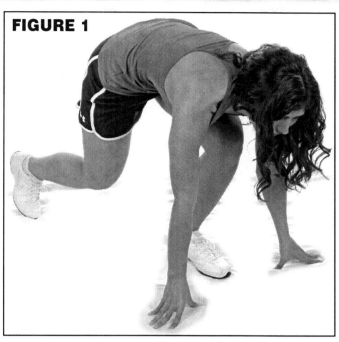

FIGURE 2

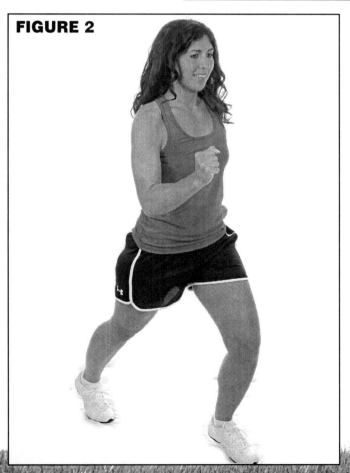

FIGURE 3

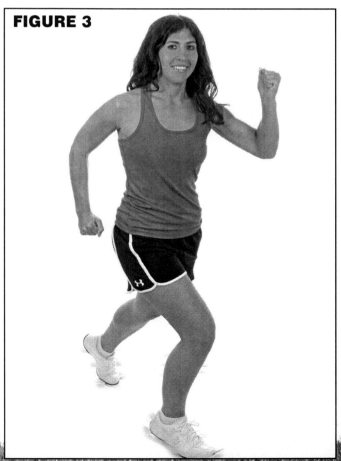

#4—CAMEL TROT

*I*magine that a cheetah and a camel decide to run a 200-mile race through the desert. The cheetah will probably jump to a quick lead. But long after the cheetah will have given up, worn out by the distance and the heat, the camel will still be striding slowly and steadily—almost rolling—over the sand to victory.

The moral of the story ladies: speed is a valuable trait, whether you are an animal, an athlete, or a mother. But for complete health and fitness, a woman needs endurance, too. After all, some days seem like a series of all-out dashes and others feel like slow-motion marathons. Practicing the Camel Trot can give you the endurance to finish even your longest days with energy to spare.

First, measure out a one-mile stretch of grass, track, or sidewalk. If you ran the Cheetah Dash on an outdoor track, you can Camel Trot there, too—a mile equals about four laps. Then, slowly and smoothly jog the distance. The object isn't to break the four-minute mile, but to maintain a slow, steady rhythm. Try to jog like the camel: roll your feet along heel-to-toe instead of slapping them down. Pounding the ground wastes energy and can cause injuries. Remember: BeautyFlex® is about training, not straining! All the "new" fitness shoes are based on our principal of the camel trot.

If running doesn't feel comfortable for you, it's no problem. Walk the distance instead, as briskly as you can without straining. Brisk walking is a healing, energizing activity—that's why doctors recommend it so highly, even for heart patients. For humans, walking is the most natural exercise there is. Give yourself the chance to move. And to enjoy moving!

SPEED, ENERGY & ENDURANCE

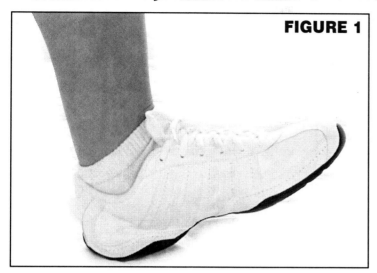

FIGURE 1

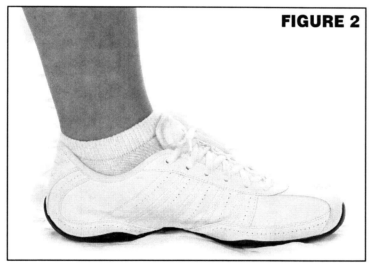

FIGURE 2

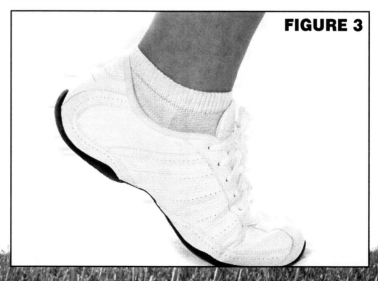

FIGURE 3

#5—CHEETAH FLEX II

*N*ow that you've climbed, dashed, and trotted, your muscles and joints are well warmed up. This last BeautyFlex® is similar to Cheetah Flex I and will stretch your legs, hips, and back to help prevent post-workout stiffness and cramping.

Stand with your feet together and your hands on your hips. Keeping your legs straight, bend forward slowly and smoothly as far as you can without straining. With both hands, try to touch the floor in front of your feet. Return to the starting position and repeat.

LEVEL THREE: 20 repetitions
LEVEL TWO: 10 repetitions
LEVEL ONE: 5 repetitions

Don't worry if you can't reach your feet, or even your ankles. When I was younger I was very stiff, and could not stretch much further than my knees, however now I can go to the floor. Remember not to bend over farther than you can comfortably. In time, your flexibility will improve.

There you go ladies. That is the workout. I would like to leave you with some last thoughts on starting your day right. As I share my heart I hope to encourage you in being consistent with your exercises.

SPEED, ENERGY & ENDURANCE

FIGURE 1

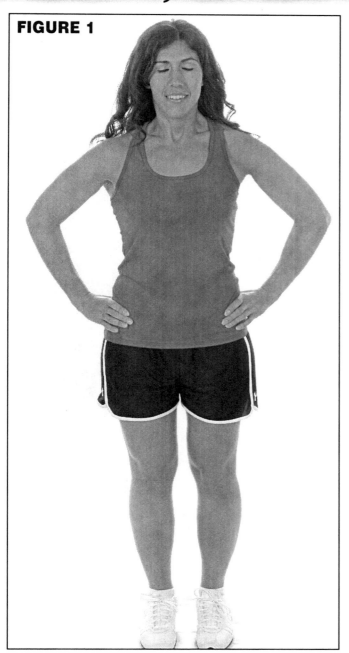

FIGURE 2

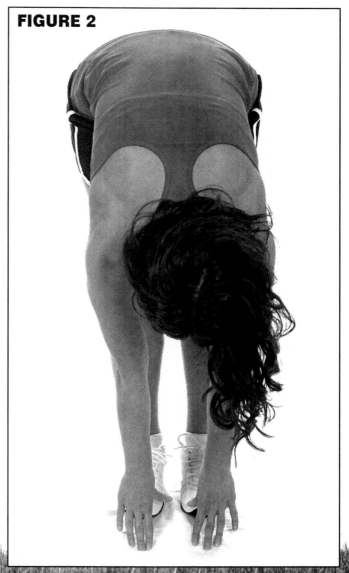

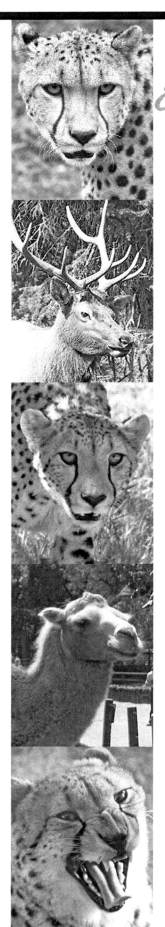

CHEETAH FLEX I

ELK CLIMB

CHEETAH DASH

CAMEL TROT

CHEETAH FLEX II

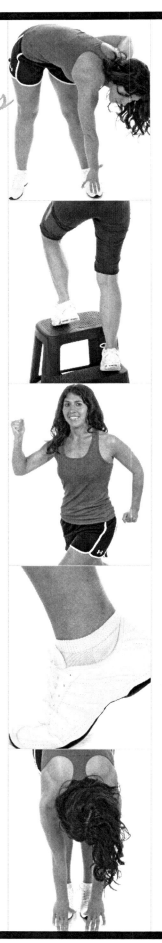

START YOUR DAY RIGHT!

*W*hether or not you are a Bible reader, I would like to share another on of my favorite verses. Philippians 4:13, *"I can do all things through Christ which strengtheneth me."*

Tap into the resources allowed for daily healing—BeautyFlex®. I do my morning stretches, spine BeautyFlexes, and immediately I start to get invigorated, and ready to take on another day.

It is the first initial movement that is the hardest You can testify to this with me, can't you? Our body wants to just sit and sulk. In our mind we know what we should do, but putting movement to the head knowledge is what is so difficult. Half the battle is beginning what we know we should do. Ladies I cannot stress the first initial movement enough. Too bad the best slogan is already taken—Just Do it! Once I just do it, I begin to feel better, I begin to limber up my body, I begin to overcome, I begin my daily healing.

I firmly believe that BeautyFlex® has been my daily dose of medicine, and healed me from a potential immobile life. Ladies, you may not have a physical ailment, but you still need to move. You still need to reap benefits from BeautyFlex®. Do not let this book sit on your shelf—tap into it everyday. Your body will thank you, as mine does on a daily basis. You will have energy, zest, and a bounce in your step that others will notice. Keep on keeping on. This is one thing that my dad always tells me, and now I am telling you all as well. You go girls!!

WRAP UP

𝒟ear Friend,

If you've followed the Workout rotation I recommended earlier in this course, you've been doing the Wild Workout® for eight weeks. During that time, you've learned and practiced 45 BeautyFlexes—All without using weights, pulleys, bars, bands, machines, or special equipment. Just like the animals you used your own body's energies and abilities to bend, twist, push, pull, flex, and move to build a brand new you! You've seen and felt what it is to work towards a goal and achieve it, But Ohhh No, you're not done yet, this is a workout for life! Whether you want to be healthy, look good, be a champion, beat out competition, or just want to stay fit. The Wild Workout® is it. Continue on and become your own best personal trainer! The Wild Workout® gives you this knowledge and the BeautyFlexes are your tools. Isn't fitness fantastic! Continue on to the end of this book and find the treasures of mix and match routines which will excel you to the next level!

I want you to have a diploma recognizing your achievement—something you can frame and look at to remind yourself of where you've come from, where you are, and where you're going. I hope you'll fill out the application on the Certificate of Achievement page and return it to me. If you like, send me a few words about your experience with Wild Workout®. It would be my privilege to rejoice with you in your success. Thank you for allowing me to share this course with you, and for allowing me to help you begin to build the body—and life—you were always meant to have.

Your Friend,

Jim Forystek

Creator, Wild Workout®

Wild WORKOUT BEAUTYFLEX

Getting to Know the Forysteks

*J*ulia Forystek attended Liberty University where she earned her degree for elementary education. She is the author of BeautyFlex and did extensive work in writing school curriculum. Julia is a certified BeautyFlex personal trainer and has been an instructor for health clubs, schools, fitness centers, and universities as well as being the head coach for girl's tennis. She also is a fitness model and educator!

Julia's Quick Workout:

Panther Flex I—10 reps
Dolphin Flex I—10 reps
Panther Flex I—10 reps
Dolphin Flex I—10 reps
Shark Flex II—20 reps
Eagle Flex I—15 reps
Bear Flex I—15 reps
Panther Flex I—10 reps
Dolphin Flex II—15 reps
Elk climb—10 reps

Julia's Hard Workout:

Panther Flex I—20 reps
Dolphin Flex II—15 reps
Panther Flex I—15 reps
Dolphin Flex II—15 reps
Panther Flex I—15 reps
Dolphin Flex II—15 reps
Eagle Flex I—20 reps
Bear Flex I—20 reps
Bull Elk Flex I—20 reps
Gorilla Flex I—20 reps
Dolphin Flex I—15 reps
Kangaroo Flex III—25 reps each leg
Frog Flex I—25 reps
Dolphin Flex III—10 reps
Cheetah Dash—5 reps
Elk Climb—10 reps

Jamee Forystek attended Liberty University where she earned her degree for exercise science and Kinesiology. She has done extensive work in physical therapy, and she is also a certified personal trainer. Jamee has been the fitness instructor for health clubs and universities as well as coaching girl's tennis and volleyball. Jamee is a fitness model and also a designer of fitness apparel. I really enjoy doing this workout to push myself to the max.

Jamee's Favorite Routine:

Panther Flex I—75 Reps (break it up sets of 25)

Dolphin Flex I—60 Reps

Dolphin Flex II—100 Reps (break it up 50, 50)

Dolphin Flex III—60 Reps

Frog Flex I—50 Reps

Frog Flex II—25 Each Direction

Elk Climb—15 Reps

Cheetah Dash—10 Reps

Cheetah Flex II—5 Reps

My Healthy Workout Snack:

2 Celery Sticks with natural Peanut Butter and

1 cup of vanilla all natural yogurt with cinnamon sprinkled on top

*B*renda Forystek is a graduate of the Barbizon school of modeling and has been a professional model doing work for print campaigns, live campaigns, and runway modeling. She is the mother of all five of the Forystek fitness animals; Julia, Jamee, Jim, John, and Jed.

Brenda's favorite routine is any length of stairs or flight of stairs indoors or out doing the BeautyFlex Elk Climb.

WILDWORKOUT® BEAUTYFLEX® ROUTINES

$\mathcal{W}$elcome to the Wild Workout® BeautyFlex® Routine Section. Here you will learn all about our Wild Workout® Routines. Starting with finding exactly what you are looking to accomplish, we'll show you how to arrive at the routine, and you can either pick from a pre-made routine, find a routine where you can add the exercises of your choice or use our approaches and routines to help build the perfect routine, as we help you to become your own best personal trainer with Wild Workout®. We understand that each person is a unique individual with different personalities, likes, dislikes, body-types, shapes, desires and goals. Here you will find many different structured routines that will get you great results, exactly what you are looking for. We will also show you how to structure you own personal routines to help you become YOUR OWN BEST PERSONAL TRAINER! You will never have to get bored of doing the same old routine over and over again! Whether you want to mix up your workout every 8 weeks, 4 weeks, weekly, or even daily with Wild Workout® BeautyFlex® we will show you how!

There are three main approaches to consider when choosing or structuring your routines. Whether you are a beginner and this is your first time ever exercising, or whether you are an avid exerciser, you can use these three routine approaches to get exactly what you want out of exercising. Whether you use each individual approach, put two together, or use all three together to have an exciting, fun Wild Workout® BeautyFlex® routine you love!

Before you start choosing and structuring your workout you must decide WHAT IS YOUR GOAL/ TARGET! It can be simple and very basic or go as detailed as you want. You can have a simple goal of you want to lose 10 pounds and get firm and tone legs and abs, or you can go more detailed and want firm and tone legs, a flat defined stomach, flab-free arms all while getting a full body workout, and doing a lot of cardio. You can decide if you want to start an 8 week routine, or just do daily routines. Define your goals whether big or small, basic or detailed. It could also be just listing your problem areas and what you want to improve. Do you want to lose weight? Do you want to be lean and tone? Is your biggest problem area in your stomach, legs, arms, back, or all of the above? Or are you just looking for a basic workout to keep you healthy and active? When it comes to Wild Workout® BeautyFlex®, through our help, YOU CAN BECOME YOUR OWN BEST PERSONAL TRAINER! After all, YOU know YOURSELF the best! Decide what you want and find the routine that best suites you and that you feel will best help you achieve your goals, or use these approaches and routines to help develop your own custom Wild Workout® BeautyFlex® routine. Remember you can start slow and work your way to where you want to be! Being fit & healthy doesn't come overnight in one day, but it's a day by day, week by week, month by month process. The key is to keep consistent week after week and also remember to keep track of what you have done, or haven't done, ate or didn't eat, and write it all in your Wild Workout® Beauty-Flex® Journal! You cannot eat an entire elephant all in one bite, but it's a bite by bite process that gets the job done. With defining your goals you can start small and work your way bigger, build your confidence and remember obtaining and maintaining a fit and healthy lifestyle is not just a one-time thing, but it is a continual choice that you'll learn to love and something you will want to do regularly because of how much joy and satisfaction you will get from it.

The first approach is the **DIRECT TARGET APPROACH**. In the direct target approach you are going to approach your exercises in full sections, exercise by exercise. If you decide you want to start your path to flat, firm, defined abs, you will take the abdominal section in one workout performing one exercise at a time resting between exercises and sets. You will concentrate specifically on that exercise until it is complete. Then you will move on to the next exercise. You can break each exercise into sets resting between each set, or do them all in one continuous set and resting between exercises. For example if want to exercise your ABDOMINALS with the Direct Target Approach you will do:

Dolphin Flex 1 (Level 1-3 Until Complete)

Short Rest (30 seconds – 3 Minutes)

Dolphin Flex 2 (Level 1-3 Until Complete)

Short Rest (30 seconds – 3 Minutes)

Shark Flex 1 (Level 1-3 Until Complete)

Short Rest (30 seconds – 3 Minutes)

Shark Flex 2 (Level 1-3 Until Complete)

Short Rest (30 seconds – 3 Minutes)

Dolphin Flex 3 (Level 1-3 Until Complete)

You may perform Level 1 through Level 3 Repetitions remembering that Level Three is for optimal performance, satisfaction, and results. Always train and never strain, if you need to start at level one, start at level one. Break each exercise up into sets as well, as you do not need to perform any exercise all in a row (unless you want to or can). For example if performing the Frog Flex I Level 3 you don't need to do 80 in a row (as many people cannot) but break them into sets. See below:

8 Sets of 10 Repetitions in a row (8x10=100)
Rest between each set (30 sec - 3 min)

4 Sets of 20 Repetitions

2 Sets of 20 Reps & 2 Sets of 15 Reps

2 Sets 40 Reps

Break them down however you feel comfortable

In the Direct Target Approach you may also be specifically targeting more than one muscle group in a single workout. For example you could work your Abdominals, Legs and Arms all in one workout in one day. Choose which section you want to start with and perform that section until complete, move onto the next section, and then the last section doing each section laid out above with the abdominal example. The Direct Target Approach is great for targeting specific muscle groups for maximum results to strengthen, develop and tone your muscles!

The second approach is the **MIX AND MATCH APPROACH.** In the mix and match approach you are going to approach your exercises by mixing and matching them into your routine to give you a creative, fun way to put your exercises together to get a great workout. In the Mix and Match Approach you do not have to perform the entire section like with the Direct Target Approach (unless you want to). For example if you want to work your abs, chest, arms, back and legs all in one workout in one day, you may not have the time using the Direct Target Approach, but with the Mix and Match approach you can choose 1-3 exercises from each section you are looking to work and put them together for a creative, unique workout routine that could look something like this.

Dolphin Flex 1 (Level 1-3 Until Complete)
Short Rest

Shark Flex 2 (Level 1-3 Until Complete)
Short Rest

Panther Flex 1 (Level 1-3 Until Complete)
Short Rest

Eagle Flex 1 (Level 1-3 Until Complete)

Short Rest

Gorilla Flex IV (Level 1-3 Until Complete)

Short Rest

Lion Flex I (Level 1-3 Until Complete)

Short Rest

Horse Flex I (Level 1-3 Until Complete)

Short Rest

Mule Flex (Level 1-3 Until Complete)

Short Rest

Frog Flex I (Level 1-3 Until Complete)

Short Rest

Frog Flex II (Level 1-3 Until Complete)

In this example you are performing 10 exercises from five different sections which would take about the same workout time as performing two sections from the Direct Target Approach.

How to use The Mix and Match Approach and the Direct Target Approach at the same time: You can easily put the Direct Target Approach and the Mix and Match Approach together in one workout by Directly Targeting one or two sections and mix and matching a couple other sections. You could directly target the Abs and Arms, while Mix and Matching the Chest, Legs, and Neck. It would look something like this:

Abs (Direct Target)	**Chest** (Mix and Match Pick 1-3)
Arms (Direct Target)	**Legs** (Mix and Match Pick 1-3)
	Neck (Mix and Match Pick 1-3)

The Mix and Match Approach is great for getting a full body workout, hitting all major muscle groups, without having to perform the entire section! Also great for fun, creative workouts that will help burn fat and tone muscle!

The Third Approach is the **CIRCUIT APPROACH**. In the Circuit Approach you are going to approach your exercises by doing them in a continuous circuit. This approach is not only great for muscle toning but **fantastic for fat burning!** *On days where you are looking for a great cardio workout and don't quite feel like doing the Speed, Energy and Endurance section and putting your running shoes* *on, do the Circuit Approach!* The Circuit Approach is an excellent, excellent cardio workout! In the Circuit Approach you will be performing one exercise right after another with no rest time in between. In this approach you will only perform one set of a particular exercise then move to the next exercise set and when you've completed one set of each selected exercise you will come back to the beginning and perform each exercise again until you reach your desired number of repetitions for those exercises. There are multiple approaches to the Circuit approach and you can find the one you enjoy the best.

For example if you want to perform the Chest and Abdominal sections (full sections like in the Direct Target Approach) you could do so using the Circuit Approach. You can do both sections, all 10 exercises in a single circuit, or do each section by itself in a circuit (5 exercises at a time) or pair them two by two.

If performing both exercises in one circuit, have a starting number that's easily obtainable for at least 2 times through the circuit. So let's say you are going to start performing each exercise for 10 repetitions. You will perform the following with NO REST. Once you complete the circuit one time through you can have a short rest (if you really need it) before performing it again. Of course, if you have to rest during the circuit, you can, just try to set your reps at a reasonable number where you will not tire yourself out too quickly. If performing two sections together in a single circuit try alternating each exercise from one section to the next section to give your muscle groups a rest so you will not tire out one muscle group too fast. (Example below)

Panther Flex I — 10 Reps

Dolphin Flex I — 10 Reps

Eagle Flex I — 10 Reps

Dolphin Flex II — 10 Reps

Bear Flex I — 10 Reps

Shark Flex I — 10 Reps

Gorilla Flex I — 10 Reps

Shark Flex II — 10 Reps

Elk Flex I — 10 Reps

Dolphin Flex III — 10 Reps

(Repeat with no rest between exercises until desired level is reached)

A good goal to set is performing through each circuit at least 3 times.

If you want to pair exercises in two's with the circuit approach you could do it this way:

> **Panther Flex I** — 10 Reps
>
> **Dolphin Flex I** — 10 Reps
>
> *(Repeat until exercise level complete)*
>
> **Eagle Flex I** — 10 Reps
>
> **Dolphin Flex II** — 10 Reps
>
> *(Repeat until exercise level complete)*
>
> **ETC...**

Using the Circuit Approach is also great with the Mix and Match Approach. You can use multiple circuits or just one. You could Mix and Match Chest, Abs, Legs, & Back choosing 1 exercise from each and putting them into a circuit that could look like this:

> **Panther Flex I** — 15 Reps
>
> *No Rest*
>
> **Dolphin Flex I** — 10 Reps
>
> *No Rest*
>
> **Frog Flex I** — 20 Reps
>
> *No Rest*
>
> **Horse Flex I** — 5 Reps
>
> *(Perform Circuit 5 Times)*

All the reps do not have to be the same for each exercise. Some exercises you may be better at and some you may need improvement. You can have a higher or lower number of reps for each exercise, and use them for your circuit. The exercises themselves do not need to be performed speedily in the Circuit Approach; it's only that there is no rest time between exercises unless absolutely necessary.

Wild Workout® BeautyFlex® Routines

During the Wild Workout® BeautyFlex® Routines remember to drink water before, during and after workouts. If you ever get exhausted; stop, rest, and drink water. Start slow and work your way up. It is advised you start with the introductory eight week program to learn all 45 different exercises and build a good foundational strength and physique for you to continue to build upon with the Wild Workout® BeautyFlex® Routines. We recommend you exercise 3-5 days per week. The following routines have daily routines in which you can pick from day to day workouts finding what routine you feel like doing that day, weekly routines, 4 week routines, and 8 week routines. Depending on your schedule, family, work, vacations, etc., we expect your exercise schedule to work around you, not you around it. With Wild Workout® BeautyFlex® You don't have to drive to the gym, you don't have to schedule an appointment, but you can exercise in the privacy of your own home, hotel, backyard, park, office, basement, bedroom, wherever you are, when it's convenient for YOU! Depending on how your routines are structured you can get great workouts lasting anywhere from 5 minutes to 1 hour.

When you see a section listed with (Direct Target) following the section, means you will do that entire section (5 exercises) via the Direct Target Approach. When you see a section listed with (Mix & Match Pick One, Two or Three) it means to pick as many exercises from that section as listed. If you see a routine listed as a Circuit Routine, use the Circuit routine approach remembering that no rest is supposed to be used between exercises. Exercises should be performed with Level One, Two or Three repetitions (Level One beginner, Level Two intermediate, and Level Three advanced).

DAILY ROUTINE — Upper Body & Core
Approach: Direct Target
Concentration: Chest, Abs, Arms

Chest (Direct Target)

Abs (Direct Target)

Arms (Direct Target)

DAILY ROUTINE — Lower Body, Core, & Cardio
Approach: Direct Target
Concentration: Legs, Abs, Speed, Energy & Endurance

Legs (Direct Target)

Abs (Direct Target)

Speed, Energy & Endurance (Direct Target)

DAILY ROUTINE — Full Body
Approach: Direct Target and Mix & Match
Concentration: Legs, Abs (Direct Target); Chest, Shoulders (Mix & Match)

Legs (Direct Target)

Chest (Panther Flex I & Pick One)

Abs (Direct Target)

Shoulders (Pick Two)

DAILY ROUTINE — Full Body

Approach: Direct Target and Mix & Match

Concentration: Chest, Back (Direct Target); Legs, Arms, Abs (Mix & Match)

Chest (Direct Target)

Arms (Pick Two)

Abs (Pick Two)

Back (Direct Target)

Legs (Pick Two)

DAILY ROUTINE — Full Body

Approach: Direct Target and Mix & Match

Concentration: Arms, Abs (Direct Target); Back, Legs (Mix & Match)

Arms (Direct Target)

Back (Pick Two)

Abs (Direct Target)

Legs (Pick Three)

DAILY ROUTINE — Upper Body, Core & Cardio

Approach: Mix & Match

Concentration: Chest, Abs, Back, Speed, Energy & Endurance

Chest (Panther Flex I & Pick One)

Abs (Dolphin Flex I & Pick Two)

Back (Horse Flex I & Pick One)

Speed, Energy & Endurance (Elk Climb & Camel Trot)

DAILY ROUTINE — Upper Body & Cardio

Approach: Mix & Match

Concentration: Chest, Shoulders, Neck, Speed, Energy & Endurance

Chest (Panther Flex I & Pick One)

Shoulders (Pick Three)

Neck (Pick Three)

Speed, Energy and Endurance (Camel Trot & Pick One)

DAILY ROUTINE — Full Body Power Workout

Approach: Direct Target and Mix & Match

Chest (Direct Target)

Abdominals (Direct Target)

Legs (Direct Target)

Arms (Mix & Match—Pick Two)

Shoulders (Mix & Match—Pick Two)

Back (Mix & Match—Pick Two)

Neck (Mix & Match—Pick Two)

Spine (Mix & Match—Pick Two)

Speed, Energy, & Endurance (Direct Target)

DAILY ROUTINE —
Fat Burning, Muscle Toning, Double Circuit

Approach: Circuit

Concentration: Full Body

Chest—Panther Flex I—10 Reps

Legs—Frog Flex I—10 Reps

Abs—Dolphin Flex I—10 Reps

Chest—Eagle Flex I – 5 Reps

Legs—Kangaroo Flex II—6 Reps (per leg)

Abs—Shark Flex II—5 Reps (each way)

(Perform 3-6 Times) (Short Rest & Water)

Speed, Energy and Endurance—Elk Climb—5 Reps

Shoulders—Gorilla Flex II—5 Reps (each arm)

Back—Horse Flex IV—5 Reps

Arms—Jaguar Flex I—5 Reps

Speed, Energy and Endurance—Cheetah Flex I—5 Reps (per side)

Shoulders—Cougar Flex II —5 Reps (each arm)

Back—Horse Flex I—5 Reps (each side)

Arms—Tiger Flex I—5 Reps (each arm)

(Perform 2-5 Times)

DAILY ROUTINE — Cardio & Strengthening
LESS THAN 10 MINUTES — TIME CRUNCH CIRCUIT
Approach: Circuit
Concentration: Chest, Abs, Legs

Chest—Panther Flex I—10 Reps

Abs—Dolphin Flex I—10 Reps

Legs—Frog Flex I—10 Reps

Abs—Dolphin Flex II—10 Reps

(Perform 3-6 times)

WEEKLY ALTERNATE DAY — FULL BODY & CARDIO
Approach Used: Direct Target and Mix & Match

Chest, Abs, Legs, & Back (Direct Targets)

Your Choice (Mix & Match)

Speed, Energy and Endurance (Mix & Match)

Day 1: Chest & Abs (Direct Target)

    Mix & Match Pick 3

    Elk Climb & Camel Trot

Day 2: Legs & Back (Direct Target)

    Mix & Match Pick 3

    Camel Trot & Cheetah Dash

(Repeat for days 3-6 Rest Day 7)

3-DAY WEEKLY — FULL BODY & CARDIO
Sunday-Tuesday-Thursday
Approach: Direct Target and Mix & Match
Concentration: Legs, Abs, Speed Energy & Endurance (Direct Target)
    Full Body (Mix & Match)

Legs (Direct Target)

Abs (Direct Target)

Arms (Mix & Match -Pick Two)

Shoulders (Mix & Match -Pick Two)

Chest (Mix & Match – Panther Flex I + Pick One)

Neck, Spine, Back (Mix & Match -Pick One)

Speed, Energy and Endurance (Direct Target)

4-WEEK ABS & CARDIO BLASTER WILDWORKOUT® ROUTINE
Approach: Direct Target, Mix & Match, and Circuit
Concentration: Abdominals & Cardiovascular
Level: Your Choice

WEEK 1

Day 1 & Day 4: Abs (Direct Target), Circuit: Panther Flex I - 15 Reps, Frog Flex I - 15 Reps, Mule Flex - 5 Reps (Perform Circuit 4 Times), Speed, Energy & Endurance (Direct Target)

Day 2 & Day 5: Circuit: Dolphin Flex I, Dolphin Flex II, Shark Flex I, Shark Flex II, Dolphin Flex III (Perform Circuit 3-5 Times), Speed, Energy & Endurance (Direct Target)

Day 3, Day 6, & Day 7: Off (Feel free to rest, or use a desired daily routine)

WEEK 2

Day 1 & Day 4: Circuit: Dolphin Flex I 10-15 Reps, Panther Flex I 10-20 Reps, Dolphin Flex II 15-25 Reps, Frog Flex I 10-20 Reps, Shark Flex I 5-15 Reps (Perform Circuit 4-6 Times) Circuit: Shark Flex II 10-20 Reps (Each Way), Elk Climb 4-6 Reps, Dolphin Flex III 15-25 Reps, Mule Flex 5-10 Reps (Perform Circuit 3-5 Times), Camel Trot

Day 2 & Day 5: Abdominals (Direct Target), Circuit: Panther Flex I – 10 Reps, Frog Flex I – 10 Reps, Gorilla Flex I – 5 Reps (Perform Circuit 3-7 Times), Speed, Energy, and Endurance (Direct Target)

Day 3, 6, 7: Off (Feel free to rest, or use a desired daily routine)

WEEK 3

Day 1 & Day 4: Camel Trot, Abdominals (Direct Target), Elk Climb

Day 2 & Day 5: Abdominals (Direct Target), Circuit: Panther Flex I – 10 Reps, Frog Flex I – 10 Reps, Elk Flex I – 5 Reps (Each Way) (Perform Circuit 3-7 Times), Speed, Energy, and Endurance (Direct Target)

Day 3, 6, 7: Off (Feel free to rest, or use a desired daily routine)

WEEK 4

Day 1 & Day 4: Abdominals (Direct Target (Suggested: Level Three)), Speed, Energy, and Endurance (Direct Target (Suggested: Level Three))

Day 2 & Day 5: Circuit: Dolphin Flex I – 8 Reps, Dolphin Flex II – 12 Reps, Shark Flex I – 5 Reps, Shark Flex II – 10 Reps (5 Each Way), Dolphin Flex III – 12 Reps (Perform Circuit 3 Times) Circuit: Panther Flex I – 15 Reps, Dolphin Flex I – 8 Reps, Dolphin Flex II – 12 Reps, Frog Flex I – 15 Reps, Shark Flex I – 5 Reps, Horse Flex I – 5 Reps, Shark Flex II – 10 Reps (5 Each Way), Dolphin Flex III – 12 Reps, Eagle Flex I – 5 Reps (Perform Circuit 3-5 Times)

Day 3, 6, 7: Off (Feel free to rest, or use a desired daily routine)

A 4-WEEK GETTING FIT, DON'T HOLD BACK WILDWORKOUT® ROUTINE
Approach: Direct Target and Mix & Match
Concentration: Total Body

WEEK 1

Monday & Thursday: Target Muscles → Chest and Abdominal

Panther Flex I – 4 sets of 10 reps; Eagle Flex I – 2 sets of 15 reps; Bear Flex I – 2 sets of 15 reps; Gorilla Flex I – 2 sets of 15 reps; Elk Flex I – 2 sets of 10 reps (5 Each Arm)

Dolphin Flex I – 2 sets of 25 reps; Dolphin Flex II – 3 sets of 25 reps; Shark Flex I – 2 sets of 20 reps; Shark Flex II – 1 set of 20 reps (Each Way); Dolphin Flex III – 3 sets of 25 reps

Tuesday & Friday: Target Muscles → Legs and Shoulders

Legs: Frog Flex I – 4 sets of 20 reps; Frog Flex II – 2 sets of 10 reps; Kangaroo Flex I – 2 sets of 15 reps; Frog Flex III – 2 sets of 10 reps; Kangaroo Flex II – 3 sets of 5 reps each leg

Shoulders: Gorilla Flex II – 2 sets of 20 reps; Gorilla Flex III – 2 sets of 20 reps; Rhino Flex I – 2 sets of 20 reps; Cougar Flex I – 2 sets of 20 reps; Cougar Flex II – 2 sets of 20 reps

Wednesday & Saturday: Cardiovascular

Cheetah Flex I – 30 Reps (15 Each Side); Elk Climb: 2 sets of 5 reps; Cheetah Dash: 6 reps; Camel Trot: One mile jog; Cheetah Flex II – 10 Reps

WEEK 2

Monday & Thursday: Target Muscles → Chest and Abdominal

Panther Flex I – 4 sets of 12 reps; Eagle Flex I – 2 sets of 15 reps; Bear Flex I – 2 sets of 15 reps; Gorilla Flex I – 2 sets of 15 reps; Elk Flex I – 2 sets of 10 reps (5 Each Arm)

Dolphin Flex I – 2 sets of 25 reps; Dolphin Flex II – 3 sets of 25 reps; Shark Flex I – 2 sets of 20 reps; Shark Flex II – 1 set of 20 reps (Each Way); Dolphin Flex III – 3 sets of 25 reps

Tuesday & Friday: Target Muscles → Legs and Arms

Frog Flex I – 4 sets of 20 reps; Frog Flex II – 2 sets of 10 reps; Kangaroo Flex I – 2 sets of 15 reps; Frog Flex III – 2 sets of 10 reps; Kangaroo Flex II – 3 sets of 5 reps each leg

Gorilla Flex IV – 2 sets of 20 reps; Lion Flex I – 2 sets of 20 reps; Tiger Flex I – 2 sets of 10 reps; Jaguar Flex I – 2 sets 10; Gorilla Flex V – 2 sets of 10 reps

Wednesday & Saturday: Target → Spine and Speed, Energy and Endurance

Spine: Eel Flex I – 2 sets of 10 reps; Eel Flex II – 2 sets of 10 reps; Alligator Flex I – 2 sets of 15 reps; Alligator Flex II – 2 sets of 10; Eel Flex III – 2 sets of 10 reps

Cheetah Flex I – 30 Reps (15 Each Side); Camel Trot: One mile jog; Elk Climb: 2 sets of 7 reps; Cheetah Dash: 7 reps; Cheetah Flex II – 10 Reps

WEEK 3

Monday & Thursday: Target Muscles → Chest and Back

Panther Flex I – 4 sets of 15 reps; Eagle Flex I – 30 reps; Bear Flex I – 30 reps; Gorilla Flex I – 30 reps; Elk Flex I – 20 reps (10 Each Arm)

Horse Flex I – 2 sets of 10 reps; Horse Flex II – 2 sets of 15 reps; Horse Flex III – 2 sets of 5 reps; Horse Flex IV – 2 sets of 5 reps; Mule Flex – 2 sets of 5 reps

Tuesday and Friday: Target Muscles → Spine and Neck

Spine: Eel Flex I – 2 sets of 10 reps; Eel Flex II – 2 sets of 10 reps; Alligator Flex I – 2 sets of 15 reps; Alligator Flex II – 2 sets of 10; Eel Flex III – 2 sets of 10 reps

Neck: Bull Flex I – 2 sets of 5 reps; Bull Flex II – 2 sets of 5 reps; Bull Flex III – 2 sets of 10 reps; Giraffe Flex I – 2 sets of 10 reps; Giraffe Flex II – 2 sets of 10 reps

Wednesday and Saturday: Cardiovascular

CIRCUIT: Dolphin Flex I – 15 Reps, Frog Flex I – 20 Reps, Dolphin Flex II – 20 Reps, Frog Flex II – 10 Reps (5 Each Way), Shark Flex II – 20 Reps (10 Each Way), Kangaroo Flex II – 15 Reps (5 Each Direction Each Leg), *(Perform Circuit 4 times)*

Cheetah Flex I – 30 Reps (15 Each Side); Elk Climb: 2 sets of 8 reps; Cheetah Dash: 8 reps; Camel Trot: One mile jog; Cheetah Flex II – 10 Reps

WEEK 4

Monday & Thursday: Target Muscles → Arms and Abdominal

Gorilla Flex IV – 2 sets of 20 reps; Lion Flex I – 2 sets of 20 reps; Tiger Flex I – 2 sets of 10 reps; Jaguar Flex I – 2 sets 10; Gorilla Flex V – 2 sets of 10 reps

Dolphin Flex I – 2 sets of 30 reps; Dolphin Flex II – 3 sets of 30 reps; Shark Flex I – 2 sets of 20 reps; Shark Flex II – 1 set of 20 reps; Dolphin Flex III – 3 sets of 30 reps

Tuesday & Friday: Target Muscles → Back and Shoulders

Frog Flex I – 4 sets of 20 reps; Frog Flex II – 2 sets of 10 reps; Kangaroo Flex I – 2 sets of 15 reps; Frog Flex III – 2 sets of 10 reps; Kangaroo Flex II – 3 sets of 5 reps each leg

Horse Flex I – 2 sets of 10 reps; Horse Flex II – 2 sets of 15 reps; Horse Flex III – 2 sets of 5 reps; Horse Flex IV – 2 sets of 5 reps; Mule Flex – 2 sets of 5 reps

Wednesday & Saturday: Cardiovascular

CIRCUIT: Panther Flex I – 10 Reps, Frog Flex I – 15 Reps, Eagle Flex I – 5 Reps, Kangaroo Flex II – 15 (5 Each Way Each Leg), *(Perform Circuit 3 times)*

Cheetah Flex I – 30 Reps (15 Each Side); Elk Climb: 2 sets of 8 reps; Camel Trot: One mile jog; Cheetah Dash: 8 reps; Cheetah Flex II – 10 Reps

AN 8-WEEK GET SUPER FIT WILDWORKOUT® ROUTINE

Approach: Direct Target, Mix & Match, Circuit
Concentration: TOTAL BODY WORKOUT
Required: Advanced WildWorkout® Training
Caution: For the extremely dedicated only!

Rest Time between sets & exercises for this routine unless otherwise noted is 30 secs-1 minute
Resistance should be 80-100%
Where you see (Direct Target Level 3) break the repetitions into the sets of your choice, remembering rest time between sets is to be 30 seconds – 1 minute

WEEK 1

Day 1 & Day 4: Chest (Direct Target Level 3), Abdominals (Direct Target Level 3), Speed, Energy & Endurance (Direct Target Level 3)

Day 2: CIRCUIT: Panther Flex I - 10 Reps, Dolphin Flex I - 15 Reps, Frog Flex I - 20 Reps, Panther Flex I - 10 Reps, Gorilla Flex I - 10 Reps, Shark Flex I - 10 Reps, Mule Flex - 5 Reps *(Perform Circuit 3 Times)*

Arms (Direct Target Level 3) Shoulders (Direct Target Level 3)

Frog Flex I – 2 Sets of 20 Reps, Frog Flex II – 2 Sets of 10 (Each Part), Kangaroo Flex I – 2 Sets of 10, Frog Flex III – 2 Sets of 10 (Each Leg), Kangaroo Flex II – 2 Sets of 10 (Each position, each leg)

Day 3: Back (Direct Target Level 3), Spine (Direct Target Level 3)

Circuit: Bull Flex I - 5 Reps, Bull Flex II - 5 Reps, Bull Flex III - 5 Reps (Each Way), Giraffe Flex I - 5 Reps (Each Way), Giraffe Flex II - 5 Reps (Each Way) *(Perform Circuit 2 Times)*

Camel Trot: Finish Goal= Less than 9 minutes (Rest 2 Minutes), Elk Climb – 2 Sets of 10 Reps, Cheetah Dash 7 Sets of 1 Rep, Camel Trot- WALK- Cool down

Day 4: See Above

Day 5: Legs (Direct Target Level 3), Abs (Direct Target Level 3), Arms (Gorilla Flex IV & Lion Flex I), Shoulders (Direct Target Level 3), Speed, Energy & Endurance (Direct Target Level 3)

Day 6: Back (Direct Target Level 3), Neck (Direct Target Level 3), Spine (Direct Target Level 3), Arms (Mix & Match Pick 3)

Day 7: Rest

WEEK 2

Day 1 & Day 3: Chest (Direct Target Level 3), Arms (Direct Target Level 3), Shoulders (Direct Target Level 3), Speed, Energy & Endurance (Level 3)

Day 2: Circuit: Frog Flex I – 25 Reps, Dolphin Flex I – 15 Reps, Elk Climb - 5 Reps, Alligator Flex I – 15 Reps *(Perform Circuit 4 Times)*

Circuit: Dolphin Flex II – 25 Reps, Eel Flex III – 10 Reps, Shark Flex II – 10 Reps (Each Way), Horse Flex I – 10 Reps (Each Side), Alligator Flex II – 10 Reps *(Perform Circuit 4 Times)*

Day 3: See Above

Day 4: Legs (Direct Target Level 3) Abs (Direct Target Level 3) Circuit: Panther Flex I – 10 Reps, Horse Flex IV – 5 Reps, Elk Flex I – 5 Reps (Each Side), Eagle Flex I – 5 Reps *(Perform Circuit 3 Times)*

Day 5: Circuit: Dolphin Flex I – 15 Reps, Dolphin Flex II – 25 Reps, Shark Flex I – 10 Reps, Shark Flex II – 12 Reps (Each Way), Dolphin Flex III – 25 Reps *(Perform Circuit 4 Times)*

Circuit: Panther Flex I – 33 Reps, Eagle Flex I – 20 Reps, Bear Flex I – 10 Reps, Gorilla Flex I – 10 Reps, Elk Flex I – 10 Reps (5 per side) (*Perform Circuit 4 times*) Speed, Energy & Endurance (Direct Target Level 3)

Day 6: Spine & Neck (Direct Target Level 3)

Day 7: Rest

WEEK 3

Day 1: Chest (Direct Target Level 3), Back (Direct Target Level 3), Circuit: Gorilla Flex III – 10 Reps (Each Arm), Tiger Flex I – 10 Reps (Each Arm) Rhino Flex 1 – 10 Reps (Each Arm), Gorilla Flex V – 5 Reps, Shark Flex I – 15 Reps, Kangaroo Flex II - 5 Reps (Each Way Each Leg) (Perform Circuit 3 Times) Elk Climb 2 Sets of 10 reps

Day 2 & Day 4: Speed, Energy & Endurance (Direct Target Level 3) Frog Flex I- 50 Reps, 30 Reps, Frog Flex II – 2 Sets of 20 Reps (Each Part)

Day 3: Chest (Direct Target Level 3) Circuit: Shark Flex I - 10 Reps, Dolphin Flex III – 20 Reps, Dolphin Flex I – 15 Reps, Dolphin Flex II – 20 Reps, Shark Flex II – 10 Reps (Each Way) (Perform Circuit 4 Times) Circuit: Horse Flex I – 5 Reps (Each Way), Gorilla Flex II – 5 Reps (Each Arm), Horse Flex II – 10 Reps, Gorilla Flex III – 5 Reps (Each Arm), Horse Flex III – 5 Reps, Rhino Flex I – 5 Reps (Each Arm), Horse Flex IV – 5 Reps, Cougar Flex I – 5 Reps (Each Arm), Mule Flex – 5 Reps, Cougar Flex II – 5 Reps (Each Arm) (*Perform Circuit 3 Times*)

Day 4: See Above

Day 5: Circuit: Panther Flex I – 20 Reps, Eagle Flex I – 15 Reps, Kangaroo Flex I – 10 Reps, Frog Flex III – 10 Reps (Perform Circuit Twice) Circuit: Dolphin Flex I – 15 Reps, Gorilla Flex IV – 10 Reps (Each Arm- Part One), Shark Flex I – 15 Reps, Lion Flex I – 10 Reps (Each Arm), Shark Flex II – 10 Reps (Each Way) (*Perform Circuit 3 Times*)

Day 6: Circuit: Panther Flex I – 15 Reps, Eagle Flex I – 10 Reps, Bear Flex I – 5 Reps, Gorilla Flex I 5 Reps, Elk Flex I – 5 Reps (5 Each Way) (Perform Circuit 4 Times), Back (Direct Target Level 3), Shoulders (Direct Target Level 3), Cheetah Flex I – 3 Sets of 10 Reps (Each Side), Elk Climb – 2 Sets of 10 Reps, Cheetah Dash – 10 Sets of 1 Rep, Camel Trot, Cheetah Flex II – 2 Sets of 10 Reps

Day 7: Rest

WEEK 4

Day 1, Day 3 & Day 5: Mix and Match: Panther Flex I – 30 Reps, Frog Flex I – 50 Reps, Panther Flex - 20 Reps, Frog Flex I – 30 Reps, Panther Flex I – 10 Reps, Frog Flex I – 20

Reps, Circuit: Eagle Flex I- 15 Reps, Bear Flex I - 13 Reps, Gorilla Flex I – 13 Reps, Elk Flex -7 Reps (Each Way) *(Perform Circuit 3 Times)* Abdominals (Direct Target Level 3), Speed, Energy & Endurance (Direct Target Level 3)

Day 2: Arms, Back, Shoulders (Direct Target Level 3)

Day 3: See Above

Day 4: Spine, Neck, Arms (Direct Target Level 3)

Day 5: See Above

Day 6: Shoulders, Back, Arms (Direct Target Level 3)

Day 7: Rest

REMINDER: Rest Time between sets & exercises for this routine unless otherwise noted is 30 secs-1 minute and Resistance should be 80-100%

WEEK 5

Day 1: Circuit: Panther Flex I – 30 Reps, Alligator Flex I – 15 Reps, Gorilla Flex I – 10 Reps, Alligator Flex II – 10 Reps *(Perform Circuit 3 Times)* Circuit: Dolphin Flex I – 20 Reps, Horse Flex I – 10 Reps (Each Way), Dolphin Flex II – 30 Reps, Horse Flex IV – 5 Reps *(Perform Circuit 3 Times)*, Camel Trot

Day 2: Chest (Direct Target Level 3), Arms (Direct Target Level 3), Shoulders (Direct Target Level 3), Speed, Energy & Endurance (Direct Target Level 3)

Day 3: Legs (Direct Target Level 3), Spine (Direct Target Level 3), Neck (Direct Target Level 3), Speed, Energy & Endurance (Direct Target Level 3)

Day 4: Chest (Direct Target Level 3), Abdominals (Direct Target Level 3); Camel Trot

Day 5: Arms, Back, Shoulders (Direct Target Level 3)

Day 6: Legs, Shoulders, Spine, (Direct Target Level 3)

Day 7: Rest

WEEK 6

Day 1: Abs (Direct Target Level 3), Legs (Direct Target Level 3), Chest (Direct Target Level 3); Camel Trot

Day 2: Legs (Direct Target Level 3), Arms (Direct Target Level 3), Shoulders (Direct Target Level 3), Cheetah Flex I – 15 Reps (Each Each), Elk Climb 1 Set of 20 Reps

Day 3: Abs (Direct Target Level 3), Back (Direct Target Level 3), Speed, Energy, & Endurance (Direct Target Level 3)

Day 4: Shoulders (Direct Target Level 3), Chest (Direct Target Level 3), Arms (Direct Target Level 3), Cheetah Flex II – 10 Reps, Cheetah Dash – 10 Reps, Camel Trot

Day 5: Abs, Back, Neck (Direct Target Level 3)

Day 6: Arms, Shoulders, Abdominals (Direct Target Level 3)

Day 7: Rest

WEEK 7

Day 1 & Day 4: Abdominals, Shoulders, Arms (Direct Target Level 3)

Day 2 & Day 5: Legs, Back, Neck (Direct Target Level 3)

Day 3 & Day 6: Chest, Spine, Speed, Energy & Endurance (Direct Target Level 3)

WEEK 8

Day 1: Abs (Direct Target Level 3), Chest, Arms, Shoulders (Mix and Match Pick 2 of each), Speed, Energy & Endurance (Direct Target Level 3)

Day 2: Mix and Match: Panther Flex I – 30 Reps, Frog Flex I – 40 Reps, Panther Flex I - 20 Reps, Frog Flex I – 30 Reps, Panther Flex I – 10 Reps, Frog Flex I – 20 Reps, Back (Direct Target Level 3), Cheetah Flex I – 15 Reps (Each Way), Elk Climb 1 Set of 20 Reps, Cheetah Flex II – 10 Reps

Day 3: Circuit: Dolphin Flex I – 15 Reps, Dolphin Flex II – 25 Reps, Shark Flex I - 10 Reps, Shark Flex II – 12 Reps (Each Way), Dolphin Flex III – 25 Reps, *(Perform Circuit 4 Times)*, Arms (Direct Target Level 3), Shoulders (Direct Target Level 3)

Day 4: Chest (Direct Target Level 3), Legs (Direct Target Level 3), Spine & Back (Mix and Match Pick 2 Each), Speed, Energy & Endurance (Direct Target Level 3)

Day 5: Chest, Arms, Shoulders (Direct Target Level 3)

Day 6: Abs, Legs, Neck (Direct Target Level 3)

Day 7: Rest

GROUP WORKOUT ROUTINE

Approach Used: Mix & Match

Total Body Workout

Want to exercise with your family, friends, or a group of people?

Try this workout!

Eagle Flex I (2 sets of 10 reps), Bear Flex I (2 sets of 10 reps), Panther Flex I (3 Sets of 10 reps), Frog Flex I (2 sets of 15 reps), Frog Flex III (10 reps per leg), Dolphin Flex I (25 reps), Dolphin Flex II (25 reps), Shark Flex I (15 reps), Shark Flex II (15 reps per side), Eel Flex III (10 reps), Mule Flex (10 Reps), Horse Flex III (10 reps), Alligator Flex I (10 reps), Rhino Flex I (10 reps per side), Gorilla Flex II (10 Reps per side), Cougar Flex I (10 Reps per side), Tiger Flex I (10 Reps per side), Gorilla Flex IV (15 reps per side), Lion Flex I (15 reps per side), Eagle Flex I (10 reps)

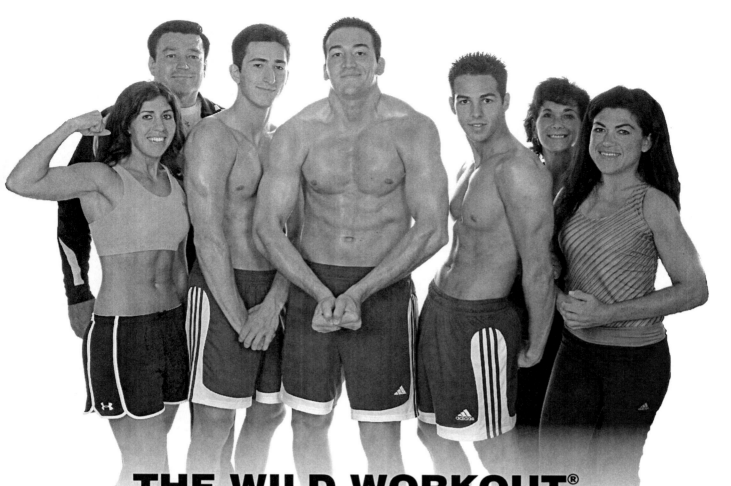

THE WILD WORKOUT®
FITNESS FOR THE
WHOLE FAMILY

PowerFlex® for the Guys of All ages
BeautyFlex® for the Girls of All ages.
Stay WILD about Working out!

www.TheWildWorkout.com

A WORD FROM DR. DWIGHT TAMANAHA

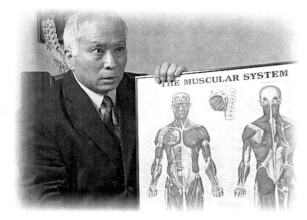

As aholistic consultant and personal trainer and a public speaker on impact-overexertion trauma, I am successfully working with amateur and professional explosive strength athletes. I find the Wild Workout® program to be one of the most effective and powerful ways to build massive amounts of muscle with maximum results in so little time! Building the normally weaker upper body region is crucial for protection against impact-overexertion trauma. The accompaniment of breathing with these exercises pushes oxygen deep into the tissues being exercised.

Dr. Dwight Tamanaha

Doctor of Chiropractic
Certified Chiropractic Sports Physician

Dr. Tamanaha is a record-holding Olympic weightlifter in his age and weight class. A former All-American and National Champion, he is published in the Southern Medical Journal, *in a medical textbook, and in the world almanac.*

QUESTIONS & ANSWERS

1. Why do Wild Workout® when I could be lifting weights instead?

*W*ild Workout® doesn't stress the spine, joints, and connective tissue with added weight, like weight-lifting does. Instead, Wild Workout® uses the body's own energy to provide resistance. It turns the body's natural movements—stretching, pulling, pushing, and flexing—into safe, healthful tools for developing strength, flexibility, power and muscle building.

I've been approached by many, many weightlifters who are dealing with chronic physical problems, including deteriorated discs and joints, torn cartilage, torn ligaments, and torn muscles. They've got bad backs, elbows, shoulders, hips, and knees. And unfortunately, many have learned to live with chronic pain.

Early on in a weightlifting workout, the muscles are still fresh enough to do the work of moving the weight. But after a few sets, once the muscles become fatigued, they're less able to support and move the weight. This means the joints, tendons, and ligaments have to do it: a surefire recipe for injury. Over time, heavy weightlifting compresses the spine, squeezing the spinal fluid out of the discs that separate the vertebrae. When there's no padding left to separate the discs, you're left with bone rubbing against bone. And pain.

2. What's the advantage of Wild Workout® over running and other forms of aerobic exercise?

*"A*erobic" means "with oxygen," and it's essential that you breathe deeply and regularly while doing your BeautyFlexes. Doing this will fill your muscles with the fresh, oxygen-rich blood that muscles need to grow and develop. Actually, all of the BeautyFlexes in this course are aerobic.

Sprinting and jogging are excellent. That's why, along with the Cheetah Dash, this course also includes the Camel Trot. However, running alone isn't enough to build complete fitness. And running long distances (longer than five miles) can, over time, cause chronic overuse injuries to the feet, ankles, knees, hips, and back similar to weight lifting problems. People whose only exercise is running long distances, or taking step aerobics or "spinning" classes, usually look healthy when they're fully clothed but since their routines don't include muscle building exercises, they may have skinny arms, narrow shoulders, and sunken chests. Maybe even flabby abs.

If you run long distances, you owe it to your long-term health to supplement your running with a low-impact, joint-friendly strength training program such as Wild Workout®.

3. Why do Wild Workout® instead of working out at a gym or a health/fitness club?

*W*ith clubs and gyms, you're paying constantly—to be taught how to use the exercise equipment, then to continue to use it. You pay for that equipment to be maintained and sanitized regularly. And for all the extras, such as juice bars and cable TV, whether you use or want them or not. If you've got a tight schedule, working out at a health club means finding time to drive to the club, paying for gas to get there and back, find a parking place, change clothes, and stand in line to use the equipment—whether the equipment has been sanitized or not.

This Wild Workout® course provides much better value for your money. It's like an owner's manual for the human body, showing you how to use your own energy and ability to sculpt your muscles, build strength, health, and add power. You can BeautyFlex® wherever you are, whenever it's convenient. You can listen to your favorite music or watch your favorite TV show. You only pay for it once, your investment will pay for itself over and over again.

4. Why BeautyFlex® instead of using one of those home gym machines?

*C*onsider the cost. Many of those treadmills, machines, gadgets, equipment and weights cost hundreds—or thousands—of dollars. And once the maintenance contract runs out—if you bought one—repair bills add to your cost.

Exercise machines are not only expensive, but they can be dangerous, too. Seats and pins break, benches collapse, and bands snap—sometimes causing serious injuries.

Thousands of these contraptions have been recalled by their manufacturers due to mechanical breakdowns (and lawsuits). On TV they always work perfectly and take up minimal floor space. But once they're delivered and set up, they're often bigger than they appear on TV. And more difficult to use. All these reasons explain why so many exercise machines become big, expensive racks to hang your old clothes on, and why so many owners give up and try to sell them, hoping to get back even a fraction of their investment.

Wild Workout® is a far better value. You're paying for a lifetime of fitness, not for big, expensive, complicated gadgets. You only pay for it once, and it's as portable as you are. You can BeautyFlex® whenever it's convenient. And best of all, Wild Workout® teaches you how to get the most out of the most brilliantly designed, incredibly functional machine you'll ever use: your own body.

5. How fit do I have to be before I can do Wild Workout®?

*W*hether you're already fit or have never exercised in your life, Wild Workout® lets you start where you are and will get you to your fitness goals, whatever they are. In no time at all you can build huge, bulging muscles and massive strength, like a gorilla, or lean, sculpted muscles with explosive power, like a panther. The more resistance you use and the higher the number of repetitions you do, the bigger your muscles will grow. With Wild Workout® achieving your fitness goals will be easy.

6. What makes Wild Workout® better than other exercise or fitness courses?

*W*ild Workout® covers every muscle in your body from head to toe and nothing is left up to guess work. Wild Workout® tell you what exercises to do, how many exercises to do, and how to do the exercises to get the body of your dreams there is no guess work or confusion. It also gives to you the ability to become your own best personal trainer, teaching you how to mix and match the BeautyFlexes to build, sculpt, and shape your muscles and also shows you how to target your problem areas that you have in your body which you never knew how to deal with to get the results that you never thought possible.

With the 45 BeautyFlexes to choose from you have such a variety that you can build completely different full body workouts of your own and never do the same routine twice, boredom from doing the same old routines are never an issue. It is truly amazing and it works, it's the Real Deal, No bull, No hype! It is all accomplished with no weights, no pulleys, no bars, no bands, no machines, no equipment, no drugs, no steroids, and no pills. It is the real deal!

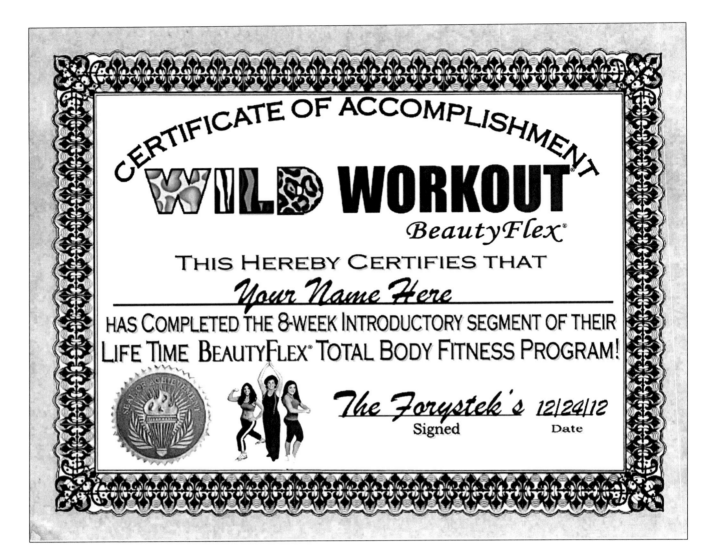

CERTIFICATE OF ACCOMPLISHMENT

*R*eceive your very own Beautiful Suitable for framing Wild Workout® diploma! Celebrate your great fitness achievement. You will want to display this beautiful diploma for all to see! You are serious about health and fitness and we would like to acknowledge your dedication.

Send a Self-Addressed Stamped Envelope to:
Forystek Fitness LLC
P. O. Box 28403
Green Bay, WI 54324

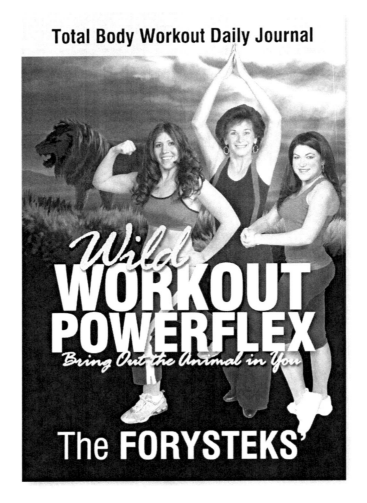

BEAUTYFLEX®

Order your BeautyFlex® Journal and DVD online at
www.TheWildWorkout.com
products page and we will ship it out to you immediately.

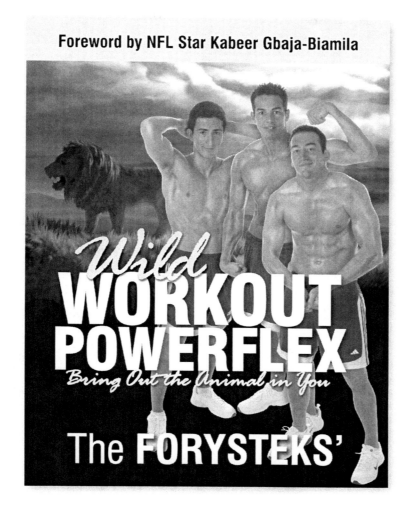

POWERFLEX®

Order your PowerFlex® Workbook, Journal and DVD online at
www.TheWildWorkout.com
products page and we will ship it out to you immediately.

CPSIA information can be obtained at www.ICGtesting.com
Printed in the USA
BVOW050416070512

289573BV00001B/10/P

9 781935 986089